Japanese Holistic Face Massage

of related interest

Vital Face
Facial Exercises and Massage for Health and Beauty
Leena Kiviluoma
ISBN 978 1 84819 166 2
eISBN 978 0 85701 130 5

Essential Oils
A Handbook for Aromatherapy Practice
Jennifer Peace Rhind
ISBN 978 1 84819 089 4
eISBN 978 0 85701 072 8

Freeing Emotions and Energy Through Myofascial Release
Noah Karrasch
ISBN 978 1 84819 085 6
eISBN 978 0 85701 065 0

Japanese Holistic
Face Massage

Rosemary Patten

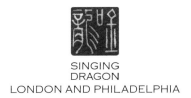

SINGING
DRAGON
LONDON AND PHILADELPHIA

First published in 2013
by Singing Dragon
an imprint of Jessica Kingsley Publishers
116 Pentonville Road
London N1 9JB, UK
and
400 Market Street, Suite 400
Philadelphia, PA 19106, USA

www.singingdragon.com

Library of Congress Cataloging in Publication Data
Patten, Rosemary.
  Japanese holistic face massage / Rosemary Patten.
    pages cm
  Includes bibliographical references.
  ISBN 978-1-84819-122-8 (alk. paper)
  1. Massage therapy. 2. Face--Massage. 3. Holistic medicine--Japan. I. Title.
  RM721.P28 2013
  615.8'22--dc23
                    2013005940

British Library Cataloguing in Publication Data
A CIP catalogue record for this book is available from the British Library

ISBN 978 1 84819 122 8
eISBN 978 0 85701 100 8

Printed and bound in China

Contents

About the Author

Rosemary Patten is a naturally gifted holistic therapist with over 23 years' experience in helping people feel better. She began her professional career within the NHS, in hospital settings, where her extensive contact with those in rehabilitation gave her an invaluable grounding in understanding the nature of disease. A master Reiki practitioner, aromatherapist, reflexologist, qualified beautician and in many other holistic therapies, Rosemary founded Rose Health and Well Being Natural Health Centre, which has now evolved into Equinox Rose. This is a combined holistic services consultancy delivering various natural therapy workshops, consultations on business development for therapists and a clinic specialising in energetic healing.

Japanese Holistic Face Massage is among the range of therapies Rosemary uses to help her many clients make a breakthrough physically or emotionally. Rosemary believes passionately in a holistic approach to diagnosing root causes of illness, especially the impact of stagnant energetic flow within and around the body.

Acknowledgements

I would like to thank the people who trusted me to help them through difficult, often heartbreaking circumstances: these brave individuals, without whose journey, which we undertook together, this book could not have been possible.

A big thank you to Jessica Kingsley – her encouraging words helped me believe in myself to do something I never thought I would be able to do. I also want to thank Lisa Driscoll and Shaileja Patel for their help with sections of this book.

I need to give a special thank you to Loreen Fraser-Owusu. Her capacity to understand and instinctively know what I wanted to express helped enormously during the draft copy-editing stages.

Last, but not least, my husband Alan, without whose unflinching support I couldn't have done this. His perceptive guidance, ability to lift my spirits when the going got tough and constant encouragement were my rock throughout this process. Moreover, without his unconditional love and belief in me over many years, I would not have been able to write this book.

Thanks to these wonderful people, I was able to affirm my intentions, bring together a comprehensive body of knowledge garnered over many years and distil that into what I hope will give the reader joy in discovering the spiritual and practical aspects of this unique massage.

Introduction

As we search for a greater truth of what life is all about, we are turning to the old ways and slowly realising our ancestors had a depth of wisdom and knowledge that in many ways surpasses that of our digital world. Our world is evolving and now a vast array of knowledge and spiritual teachings is being revealed to us. This new knowledge is coming to us so that we can make radical changes in order to save ourselves and our ailing planet from extinction. It is manifesting in an increasingly tangible cosmic shift as more and more people question their existence, turn their backs on material obsessions and look to more noble pursuits.

This spiritual and cosmic shift and the growing understanding of universal laws are essential for empowering the personal development of humankind in a way that will bring us back in tune with our true source – the universal life force. Many of these teachings would have taken years of training in the development of spiritual awareness. But, with time rapidly running out, we are being guided towards discovering this crucial knowledge, especially the understanding of the way energy flows, what energy is and how we as human beings benefit from it for our greater health and spiritual well-being.

Focusing on the old teachings of masters and sages helps us to value the importance of life as a whole – as opposed to the often insular and individualistic way we currently live in the modern world. As beings living in a world that is ever-evolving, having knowledge of these old ways is crucial to our well-being and happiness. Understanding the old teachings about the universe helps to ground us in nature and rekindle the wonder of the Divine. I cannot emphasise enough how essential this is to our survival as a species.

1

The Beginning of Time

Many ancient cultures believe in a flow of vital healing energy, within and outside the body, which rejuvenates, renews and rebalances us. This energy allows us to feel at our best regardless of what age we are. Over the centuries we have learned how to utilise this force for the good of humankind. Many assume that the origin of this idea is in Eastern philosophy, unknown to other parts of the world; however, it is universally recognised and practised by many nations across the world: from the native North American Indians, the Celts in Europe, the Aborigines of Australia, the Sufi mystics in the Middle East and Africa, to the far reaches of India and the Far East. This vital life force energy is known in Japan as Ki, in China as Qi and in India as Prana. Some people believe that the Christians' concept of the Holy Spirit is also based on this understanding of energy.

What is this energy? Simply put, it is the very essence of life: a pure energy that resonates at different levels or octaves. This healing energy is a vibration and a cosmic light that is found throughout the universe. It operates in perpetual motion, flowing around the universe, inside and around the earth. It also flows in and around all life on earth; plants, animals and even minerals process this. If there is no life force, there is no life. When the flow is impeded, there is decay and stagnation, and life ceases to exist. It's a bit like our relationship with the sun: if our sun dies, everything on earth would die with it.

HOW DOES IT AFFECT US?

An accumulation of excessive negative energy within or around the world will cause radical change to our beautiful planet, resulting in decay. Over recent centuries, through trying to dominate nature and disregarding its power, and through an increasing reliance on technology and the pursuit of amassing material possessions, we have forgotten to respect all forms of life in our quest to 'succeed'. Our abuse of it means the planet has not been able to rejuvenate and heal itself the way it should. Global warming and recent ecological disasters around the planet prove that the planet is in decay.

Stagnation of the human mind, body and soul can be caused by anything from negative belief systems, over-reliance on religion, genetic traits, environmental forces, lifestyle and our past life experiences. When we let go of past hurts and treat our body with the care and love it needs, which includes a respect for and understanding of nature, then the vital life force energy can flow freely. Physical and spiritual decay and stagnation is replaced by regeneration, harmony and vitality, ultimately restoring our vibrational resonance and giving us a feeling of optimum health, peace and enlightenment.

A NATURAL ORDER

The human race is part of a natural order connected to nature. Humans, flora and fauna are constantly changing and evolving, flowing from flux to growth. Humans have evolved at a faster rate than their co-inhabitants on earth and therefore feel superior. This has led to an increased disconnection from nature and thus a disconnection from the universal life force.

While being pure, the universal life force, or Ki, also has a duality – a negative and positive charge, or masculine and feminine trait. These two opposing forces are in effect a magnetic field consisting of a negative vibration and a positive vibration that attract and repel each other. It is known across the world by different names: the ancient Egyptians called it Nekhbet and Uatchet, the Yogi of India called it Ida and Pingala, and in China, Japan and around the Far East it is known as Yin and Yang.

According to the Hindi of India, the gods Shiva and Shakti are two opposing forces. Shakti is the creator of the earth, while Shiva is the deep consciousness or our divine potential. They are locked in an eternal embrace, dancing the dance of pleasure (Shakti) and intellect (Shiva), antagonising each other but equally in need of one another. I find this a beautiful and colourful way to describe the negative and positive energy underpinning the development of the human race.

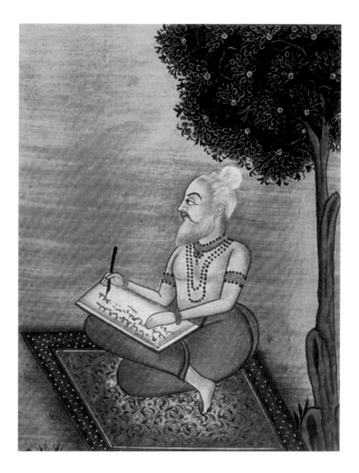

HINDU IMAGE

When vibrations within us or around us are heavy, we can attract negative energy, which makes it difficult for positive Ki energy to flow. This negative vibration can lead to feeling sluggish and possible ill health, and can be exacerbated by low moods or fatigue caused by anxiety or stress.

Everything we do and think influences us physically, mentally, emotionally or spiritually. Over our soul's many lifetimes, a vibrational imprint develops which can either support or hinder us from moving forward on our life's journey. When we allow pure celestial energy in our lives, our Ki energy within us helps to improve our outlook and physical health. Our life experiences give us an accrual of knowledge to enable our growth, which includes being able to guide others in their quest for improved resonance and well-being.

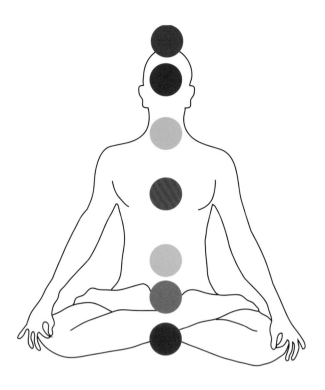

SEVEN CHAKRAS

WHEELS OF LIFE

The universal life force energy is believed to enter the body through chakras (Sanskrit meaning wheels). A chakra is a metaphoric wheel or vortex that spins and vibrates within the body. There are seven major wheels or chakras transmitting bio-energy along the spine before it is distributed further into the body via pathways and by channels or meridians (there is more about meridians on page 21). The chakras transmit the dual forces of universal life force energy, also known as 'earth's energy', comprising the feminine mother earth which is nurturing and the divine masculine which brings enlightenment.

The lower three chakras are the base chakra, sacral chakra and solar plexus. These three chakras deal with survival, pleasure and motivation. In order for us to move forward spiritually, these have to be in alignment. When they are aligned, we tend to have a love of nature and a joy of life. This alignment inspires confidence and drives us forward in a positive way towards our destiny. The heart chakra is our link between the Divine and earth. It sets us on our path to enlightenment and teaches us about compassion and unconditional love. The throat chakra deals with our interpretation of the subtle yet powerful energy that is universal law. We have now gained access to collective ancient knowledge, through listening and speaking via our connection with our higher self and the universe. The Third Eye chakra is known as the 'seat of the soul', a higher vibration, and is about knowing rather than hoping – a feeling deep inside our minds, assessing and acting on that knowledge deep into consciousness, the gateway to the Divine. The Crown chakra is a pure energy which brings us back to our spiritual source at one with the Divine.

THE BREATH OF LIFE

Our physical body depends on universal life force energy (Ki) flowing within the body. When Ki flows, the blood circulates efficiently, the digestive system works as it should and everything is in balance. Without Ki, we do not exist as it is the very breath of life.

There are five main functions of Ki: movement, transformation, protection, warming and containment. When there is Ki disharmony, the resulting imbalance is described as 'deficient Ki'. Vitality will be low and there is a feeling of tiredness and even breathlessness. 'Stagnant Ki' is when the flow is blocked, possibly through injury, emotional pain, deeply repressed feelings or anger. This will present itself in the form of mood swings, premenstrual tension, digestive problems, depression or problems with the throat. 'Rebellious Ki' is the name given when Ki flows in the wrong direction, causing coughing, belching and even vomiting.

A COMPLEMENTARY POLARITY OF OPPOSITES

The concept of Yin and Yang centres on a law of action and consequence, a duality of energetic flow. Universal energy is a constantly evolving, never static interaction between two opposing forces: a masculine downward spiral from the heavens and a feminine upward surge from the earth.

Understanding this interaction provides an awareness of people and their place in the natural order of the universe. As already mentioned, when this bio-energy or Ki is flowing freely through the body, everything is in harmony and we are one with nature and the universe. Our physical, mental, emotional and spiritual self will sing.

Yin is typically feminine, soft, wet and dark. Yang is masculine, hard, dry and light. Yin and Yang are often likened to the shady and sunny side of a hill; both have their benefits. Yin is the physical body – the cells, tissues and fluid – while Yang is the dynamic moving force of mind, spirit and intention. This concept of duality comes from the Taoist (Chinese) philosophy, first recorded by the Yellow Emperor around the third century BC, that still rings true today in our digital society.

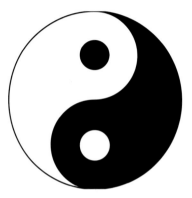

YING-YANG SYMBOL

The Yin-Yang symbol is recognised throughout the world. It is a powerful tool and illustrates in detail without words, explaining the ebb and flow of the universe perfectly.

- The circle symbolises wholeness – a never-ending cycle of Ki energy.

- A flowing line represents the change that can happen at any moment as Yin flows into Yang and Yang flows into Yin.

- There is a small dot of the opposing colour within the main colour, revealing that Yin cannot exist without Yang, like a seed that is waiting to germinate.

- There is a unique balance of equal proportions – two opposite blocks of colour with a wave that explains that life is always going to change. It will never remain static and there is a myriad of complexities between these two dynamic opposing forces.

THE ELEMENTS – A GLOBAL CONCEPT

Over centuries, many ancient civilisations have recognised parallels between nature and the physical, psychological and spiritual attributes of people. This isn't solely an Eastern concept. The Greek physician Hippocrates, the herbalist Galen, the Taoists of China, the Celtic Druids, astrologers and sages across the globe all understood the existence of a powerful force that can be used for health and the good of humankind. These attributes were grouped like the seasons and are divided into five elements or phases: Wood, Fire, Earth, Metal and Water.

The Five Phases provide a more in-depth way of describing the flow of Ki energy, especially the way it operates as a creative cycle of purity allowing for balance, with no one element dominating the other.

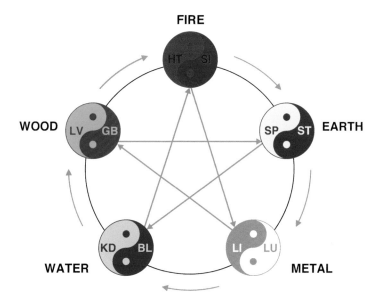

THE FIVE PHASES

THE FIVE PHASES OR ELEMENTS
'A continuous cycle'

- **Wood** – the first burst of spring's energy, the beginnings, Yang energy rising.

- **Fire** – the climax to spring, Yang energy in full glory in the summer (heat), the pinnacle, abundance and joy.

- **Earth** – the very thing that holds the four phases together, neutral, balancing interchange.

- **Metal** – the autumn or fall, keeping the most precious, contraction of Yang energy giving way to Yin, internal development (dryness), contemplation.

- **Water** – a time of recharging, old Yin regenerating, giving life, nourishing, awaiting the rebirth.

Table 1.1 The Five Phases

Element	Wood	Fire	Earth	Metal	Water
Season	Spring	Summer	Late summer	Autumn	Winter
Climate	Heat	Heat	Damp	Dryness	Cold
Yang organ	Gallbladder	Small intestine	Stomach	Large intestine	Bladder
Yin organ	Liver	Heart	Spleen	Lung	Kidney
Sense organ	Eyes	Tongue	Mouth	Nose	Ears
Body tissue	Sinews	Blood vessels	Muscles	Skin	Bone
Emotion	Anger	Joy/shock	Worry	Sadness	Fear
Colour	Green	Red	Brown	Grey	Blue
Taste	Sour	Bitter	Sweet	Spicy	Salty

The Five Elements represent a cycle of creation which also has a restraining effect and a 'natural order'. One regulates the other; for example, Fire melts Metal, Metal contains Wood by cutting, Earth allows less gravity by diminishing its pull, and Water extinguishes Fire. Thus there is a natural rhythm of one element blending into the other.

This is a simple way to understand the attributes of Ki energy, a straightforward display of the subtle vibrational differences in the flow of bio-energy. It is a vital tool that is used in diagnosis of disease within Chinese Traditional Medicine (CTM) and gives an accurate reading of possible causes of illness.

MERIDIANS
Like a river flowing down a channel

Ki flows through channels or pathways called meridians in a continuous cycle of energy. It takes 24 hours to complete the circuit flowing from lungs to liver. Where the energy is most concentrated, an organ is formed, dividing the Ki life force into qualities or aspects of Yin and Yang.

Each organ is either masculine or feminine and has the characteristics of one of the Five Elements or Phases. Each organ also has a restraining partner that complements it – for example, when you treat the small intestine (Yang) meridian, you are also treating the heart (Yin) meridian.

There are also two extraordinary channels that control the flow of Yin and Yang into the body: the Conceptual vessel controls the flow of Yin (feminine) and the Governing vessel controls the flow of Yang (masculine). The triple heater or burner, although not an organ, is vital in its function to control movement of bodily fluids, including the blood circulation and the transformation Ki energy. It is split into three sections and controls fluid and bio-energy around the upper, middle and lower areas of the body.

There are a total of 14 standard meridians, 12 relating to the organs and two relating to inward flow of Ki energy. The meridian channels are invisible to the human eye, but with practice it is possible to feel through various points (acupressure or tsubo) found along the pathways.

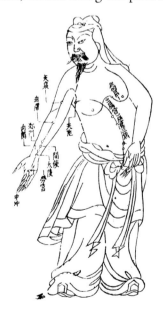

MERIDIANS AND ACUPRESSURE POINTS

POOLS OF EMOTION

Eastern medicine is based on an understanding that we are complex beings with many needs and aspirations. The ancient Chinese believed that there is a relationship between the physiology and pathology of the human body. Over time, pools of emotion gather within acupressure (tsubo) points close to the surface of the skin. Here we have easy access to the meridians to balance, regenerate and correct the flow of Ki healing energy.

ACUPRESSURE POINTS

It is an instinctive reaction to rub an area of pain for instant relief, such as rubbing the temples at the onset of a headache. It is now known that acupressure points, together with massage, can stimulate the release of endorphins within the brain. Endorphins, in a sense, are our natural painkiller. The use of acupressure is a precursor of good health as it allows the body to start the healing process. Older than acupuncture, it is believed to have been developed in India around the fifth century BC and then in China around the third century BC, spreading to Japan and the rest of the Far East.

Acupressure is effective in the treatment of physical ailments, emotional problems and improving spiritual awareness. These points correspond to organs and emotional centres within the body. Each individual point can affect the flow of Ki, and when used in a particular sequence, there is greater intensity. The practice of this ancient art has been proven to release endorphins which can ease pain, relax muscles, reduce stress and tension and boost the immune system.

Much of our knowledge of acupressure points is now being researched and is fast becoming scientific fact. Acupressure points are often located at the point of origin or insertion of the muscle. The action of stimulating certain acupressure points has a direct effect, a reflex action straight to the brain and spinal cord and to the corresponding organ.

The brain has the facility to override normal function to protect muscles from fatigue. However, due to tension or overwork, the brain continues to send impulses to maintain tension, even if the problem has abated. Acupressure points are known to decrease these impulses, allowing the muscle to recover and return to normal function. There is an improvement in the overall mood as messages to the brain are corrected and painful areas are improved. Muscles recover their normal function as the pain pathways are cleared.

The benefits of acupressure include:

- releasing muscle tension

- aiding circulation

- promoting the immune system

- reducing tension and stress

- helping to rebalance energy within the body

- enhancing spiritual awareness.

A DIAGNOSTIC TOOL

Emotional and physical function of the meridians has been used as a diagnostic tool of Chinese Traditional Medicine since the time of the Yellow Emperor. The prevailing belief was that if there is a physical dysfunction, then there must be an emotional cause. This may seem simplistic as there is usually more than one dysfunction. However, in most instances, finding the emotional root cause will aid the physical healing process and help to prevent the recurrence of any other related problems.

Having this insight enables the assessment of the dominant feature of a 'dis-ease' or disorder. Understanding the interaction of the Five Elements in relation to the body's physiology and its emotional state also greatly enhances the effectiveness of a treatment.

IN A NUTSHELL

- A vast array of knowledge and spiritual teaching is being made available to us to reconnect our understanding of the delicate balance between nature, the universe and the Divine.

- The flow of universal life force energy is understood throughout the world to be essential to our existence on earth. It is the very essence of life. A pure, healing energy with a polarity of opposites, it flows in and around all life on earth – plants, animals or minerals. Without it, we would cease to exist.

- Ki energy is split into Five Elements, comprising Wood, Fire, Earth, Metal and Water.

- The Five Elements is a global concept and is a simple representation of the cycle of creation. It not only describes the seasons but also helps us to understand the way Ki flows in and around the body.

- Ki energy has feminine or masculine aspects or qualities – Yin and Yang.

- Ki energy flows through channels or pathways called meridians. There are 14 standard meridians that enable a continuous flow into organs and extraordinary vessels. The meridians are accessible through acupressure points.

- The flow of Ki energy and the meridians help to explain the relationship between the physiology and pathology of the human body.

- Acupressure points enable effective treatment of physical, emotional and spiritual imbalances by regulating the flow of Ki.

- Understanding the interaction of the Five Elements in relation to the body's emotional and physiological state serves as a very useful diagnostic tool.

2

History

The Japanese have the ability to take the best from other cultures and make it their own, while still maintaining a way of life that sets them apart. Their strength of character has remained, despite Japan being relatively small in size compared to its powerful neighbours, Russia and China.

Japan's past was rooted in folklore and its ancient religion, Shinto, before monks from Tibet and India founded Buddhism around 4000 BC as the dominant religion. Along with their way of life, the Buddhist monks also brought massage to Japan.

In addition, there was an influx of people from China, bringing with them the philosophies of Taoism and Confucianism, together with their advanced knowledge of medicine, including acupressure, skills in herbalism, a unique approach to diagnosing illness, and, later, acupuncture.

As long ago as the third century BC, the Chinese courtesans used a form of rejuvenating face massage which included the application of acupressure points. The empresses of China, who had a beauty that was highly regarded, would use this treatment as part of their beauty routine which gave them luminous, clear and glowing skin. As well as looking good on the outside, this beauty regime helped them to maintain serenity on the inside while promoting physical health and longevity. A non-invasive treatment, this was a secret weapon in the empresses' quest for power, known only to a few and passed down from master to master.

There was a period of self-imposed isolationism during the Edo reign under the rule of the Tokugawa Shogunate (1603–1868) which allowed the Japanese to develop their own style of Chinese Traditional Medicine (CTM), handed down from master to student. The use of acupuncture was restricted to members of the nobility. Massage and acupressure became the accepted practice for health within Japan, although there was some Western influence from the Dutch. Eventually, massage became a profession for the blind, which restricted its development, creating a divide and leading to massage being viewed as having a lower status. In contrast, within China massage maintained an equal status alongside acupuncture and herbalism.

Massage known as amna (Japanese for massage) and tsubo (acupressure points) were associated with relaxation and pleasure – an art form. Massage was open to individual interpretation by various masters, leading to different styles of practice. During the late nineteenth century and early twentieth century there was a resurgence of interest in the benefits of massage and acupressure for medicinal purposes, including the development of a new form of massage known as Shiatsu.

JAPANESE FACE MASSAGE

Japanese face massage combining amna and tsubo became increasingly popular during the eighteenth and nineteenth centuries. It became a particular favourite with the Geisha as it promoted longevity and helped to reflect inner calm on their porcelain-like faces. The knowledge of this unique massage was not really known in the West until after the Second World War.

You are about to experience an introduction to Japanese Holistic Face Massage (JHFM). Unlike Western face massage, this massage works on all levels: physically stimulating, mentally relaxing, emotionally calming and spiritually uplifting.

Without a doubt, there are tangible differences between Western massage styles and those of the East. Western massage predominantly tends to focus on improving the circulation of blood flow and the lymphatic system. The aim of physical manipulation is to release toxins, remove dead cells and bring nourishment to a specific area in order to attain a better complexion and toned muscles. Many facials are reliant on the use of products that are artificially produced in a laboratory rather than evolved through processes in nature. Some invasive techniques designed to enhance a person's beauty can have bad side effects. Japanese massage is more exacting and has stood the test of time. The techniques focus more deeply to achieve more effective results. This is largely because of the non-invasive nature of tsubo (acupressure points) and the process of balancing Ki in the techniques used. This massage stimulates and regenerates cells within the body, bringing a lustre to the skin and an inner glow of calm and vitality. It is a complete health system of beauty and health.

While in the West we spend thousands of pounds trying to look good with the latest products or surgical techniques, the Eastern philosophy of beauty centres on inner beauty, having a quiet mind and a spiritual purpose achieved by balancing Ki. Eastern traditions of perfection are based on a belief in an afterlife and not on material wealth in this life. To be beautiful in Japan means to be healthy, radiant and spiritually grounded.

The Japanese idea of a beautiful face has been perfected by understanding the complexity of a system of medicine that existed long before the Western concept of medicine evolved. Theirs was a system based on massage and acupressure (acupuncture was added later), knowledge of meridians or energy channels, and a process of rejuvenating universal life force energy (or bio-energy) within the body.

The Japanese concept of health and well-being is based largely on preventing 'dis-ease' through self-awareness, monitoring emotional and spiritual health, and modifying the mind should any negative feelings pervade, rather than tackling and treating illness once it sets in.

A REFLECTION OF THE TRUE YOU

The face reflects who we are, our personality, our state of health and our spiritual balance. We pick up a lot of information about a person just by looking at their face. Traditional Chinese practitioners and later the Japanese knew how important the flow of Ki energy around the face was and developed how to read faces and release blocked Ki in order to bring about harmony. To the ancient Japanese and Chinese, a beautiful face was the ultimate prize because it was a reflection of optimum health – and, of course, with good health comes a long life. Longevity achieved through preventing ill health was the aim of Chinese Traditional Medicine.

IN A NUTSHELL

- Japan has a rich and diverse culture which has evolved over the centuries.

- Key phases in Japan's history, such as the Edo reign and the influx of the Chinese and their philosophies and ideologies, have helped shape its culture as we know it today.

- These notable phases also played a huge part in the evolution of massage in the country.

- The Japanese believe in beauty as the ultimate prize of good health, and massage is essential to this.

- Faces hold the key to a person's personality and their state of health, mind and spirit.

- The flow of Ki energy around the face is used to diagnose state of health.

3

The Power of Touch
Anatomy and Physiology

AN INSTINCTIVE REACTION to emotion – the squeeze of someone's hand, a warm engulfing hug, a soft caress, these say 'I understand', 'I support you', a union of two people within a second, a connection of pure love simultaneously felt. This is the power of touch.

The sense of touch develops first in the embryo and is an instinctive action between primates, who thrive on touch. Massage is one of the most ancient of therapies and triggers the release of endorphins to relax and calm the body. The skin is the largest organ of the body and performs many functions including temperature control, holding internal organs in place and protecting the body from pathogens invading it. It goes without saying that we need to look after our skin.

A CONCEPT OF HEALTH

The Japanese believe in beauty as the ultimate prize of good health. Over the centuries, massage has played an important part in maintaining that philosophy.

Eastern philosophy and health centres around prevention, a healthy lifestyle, respect for the body, expanding the mind and being in touch with the higher self.

It is no coincidence that the Japanese have perfected a form of massage that not only maintains a beautiful face but also flushes out toxins and releases emotional tension. When performed correctly, this massage even teaches recipients to bypass their ego so they can connect with their higher self, thus healing on a spiritual level.

I feel very strongly that JHFM should be universally known in order to treat as many people as possible for many different reasons.

MASSAGE TECHNIQUES

The Eastern approach to massage is more diverse than Western massage. The Eastern method comprises deep tissue manipulation to loosen tired muscles, light movements to stimulate lymphatic flow and application of light pressure to the meridians to improve the flow of Ki. The result is a truly holistic experience that refreshes and rebalances the mind, body and spirit.

Japanese Holistic Face Massage incorporates effleurage, stretches, tapotement and petrissage within the opening and closing movements. Below is an explanation of what each facet of the opening movements is all about.

EFFLEURAGE MOVEMENTS

These are slow, smooth, rhythmic stroking movements that follow the contours of the face and neck. Their key function is warming the area.

The light stroking movements result in a reflex action from the skin, improve circulation, help to remove lymphatic waste and renew the skin cells via the lymphatic system from the surface of the skin.

The application of deeper effleurage releases tense muscles, drives the removal of lactic acid and toxins, and improves the surface of the skin by limiting blemishes. This ultimately leaves the skin feeling soft and supple.

TAPOTEMENT MOVEMENTS

This is a light rhythmic tapping performed by the finger-pads after the muscles are relaxed and is essentially a type of petrissage. This action of rhythmic compression and relaxation of the muscles further increases lymphatic activity, releasing any toxins that may have built up. It stimulates cell regeneration by flooding the area with oxygen and providing nutrients to the skin surface and muscles.

PETRISSAGE MOVEMENTS

The petrissage technique is a stronger and deeper compression movement that includes thumb kneading, rolling and lifting of the skin and muscles, which promotes vascular stimulation and leaves muscles relaxed.

IMPROVED COLLAGEN AND ELASTIN EFFICIENCY

The stimulation of the circulation and blood increases the metabolic rate, which in turn supports the renewal of cells. There is an increased efficiency of collagen and elastin, making the skin feel more supple and nourished. The colour and texture of the skin are improved, creating a healthy and smooth complexion.

LYMPHATIC FLOW

Many of the acupressure points are connected to lymph nodes (see below), which further highlights the value of activating these points. Doing so stimulates and improves the flow of nutrients and oxygen to the area. Toxins and cell waste are released back into the bloodstream before being flushed out of the body altogether. An efficient lymphatic system helps to maintain a clear complexion, improves the metabolism of the skin and makes the skin feel firmer. This prevents a build-up of facial fluid and lessens puffiness on the face.

LYMPH

The lymph is a straw-coloured fluid which flows through a network of minute channels. Lymph fluid bathes muscles and skin tissue in nutrients. The waste material is then filtered into chambers or nodes where microscopic foreign particles, including pathogens and cell debris, are filtered, while the white cells destroy any invaders before the lymph rejoins the main bloodstream.

The movement of lymph is reliant on muscular activity. Sluggish or tense muscles can lead to a build-up of lymph, causing the face to become puffy, especially around the eyes.

Massage encourages lymph to flow, and many of the acupressure points within JHFM are near to or found directly resting on lymph nodes.

MUSCLE EFFICIENCY

The JHFM routine also enables direct contact with the origin and insertion (see page 37) of the facial muscles. Through these points, Ki energy is activated where it is needed: direct to the muscles. The use of acupressure and tracing of the meridians improves the contour of the face, tones the muscles and diminishes the appearance of fine wrinkles. It is a truly non-invasive beauty routine that helps to re-educate the muscles to work more efficiently.

RELEASING MUSCLE TENSION

Efficiency of connective tissue and muscles is achieved by improving the flow of lymph and elimination of toxins. This aids efficiency in circulation and allows renewal to take place. Ki energy input to the muscles is facilitated by the massage of acupressure points and the tracing of meridians.

UNDERSTANDING THE FUNCTION AND FORMATION OF SKIN

The skin is formed of the epidermis (topmost layer), the dermis (middle layer) and the subcutaneous tissue, which is the deepest layer composed of fat cells and connective tissue.

The skin's primary functions include:

- Protection of internal organs from injury and providing a protective barrier from chemical and bacterial damage for the delicate structures within.

- Synthesis of vitamin D.

- Sensory nerves – our sense of touch – within the top layers (epidermis) allow us to react to pain and pressure, detect changes in the environment in order to regulate body temperature, excreting sweat from glands to cool the body, while fat stored within the dermis and subcutaneous layers acts as insulation.

- The sebaceous glands within the epidermis secrete sebum which, together with sweat, forms the acid mantle (see Chapter 4) and maintain the skin's suppleness.

- A form of communication through blushing or excessive sweating; letting people know what emotions a person may be feeling.

- The excretion of salts and small amounts of waste such as ammonia and urea through sweat.

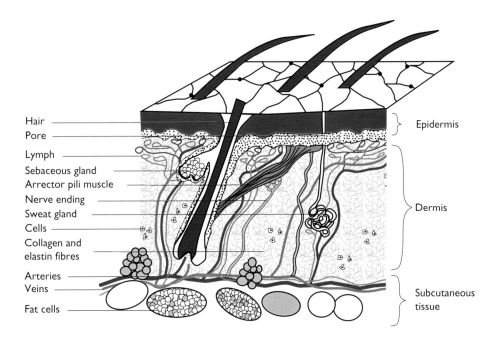

THE STRUCTURE OF THE SKIN

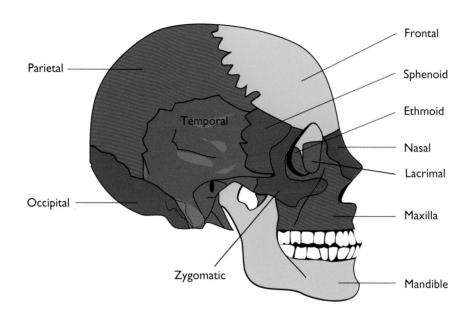

THE CRANIUM

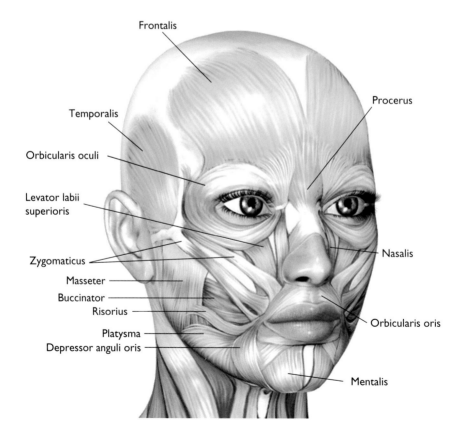

THE MUSCLES OF THE FACE

UNDERSTANDING THE MUSCLES OF THE FACE AND NECK

The facial muscles are a complicated network of sensory and motor nerves that attach to the facial bones by tendons. The structure of the face varies from person to person and depends on individual bone structure, genetic inheritance and age, giving each person their own unique appearance. The superficial facial muscles of expression and mastication have a profound influence on the outer contours of the face and the skin's appearance.

Skeletal or voluntary muscles are known as striated, due to the characteristics of individual muscles forming cylindrical cells, called fibres. The cells lie parallel to one another and, when examined closely under a microscope, look like bands of dark and light fibres. These fibres bundle together to form a fleshy mass, while the extensions of fibres, or tendons, attach to the bone or each other. The point of attachment where there is resistance is known as the origin of the muscle as it remains static, while the point of release as the muscle lengthens is called insertion.

Movement is achieved by the contraction and relaxation of individual muscles or groups of muscles or their tendons. As one muscle relaxes, the corresponding muscle contracts, thereby causing the relaxed muscle to stretch. The stretching muscle is known as the antagonist. A muscle is never completely in a relaxed state because some fibres remain partially contracted. This is known as muscle tone.

Applying massage to the muscles helps prevent muscle fatigue and works deep into the muscle fibres to stimulate the dermis. This also renews the elasticity in the top layer (epidermis), leaving the skin, smooth and firm.

NERVOUS SYSTEM

Our body is a wonderful machine that processes everything that happens externally and internally, making adjustments as needed. When the body is functioning correctly, it will respond appropriately to changes in the environment in order to keep us safe and healthy. Our sensory nerves, for example, register changes in touch, temperature and pain, and send messages to the brain which helps the body respond accordingly. The central nervous system (CNS) is the processing centre for these functions and mainly consists of the brain and the spinal cord.

AUTONOMIC NERVOUS SYSTEM

The autonomic nervous system (ANS) divides into two sections: the sympathetic nervous system, which deals with our response to danger, and the parasympathetic nervous system, which handles the regular functions of our bodies such as digestion of food. These two systems work together for our survival.

The sympathetic nervous system allows us to move out of the way of danger – commonly known as 'fight or flight'. Our ability to act quickly is vital to our survival as a species; however, in many people it has now become overactive, creating problems.

The reflex action is our instinctive, unconditioned response to changes in our environment or changes arising within the body – for example, taking preventative steps to get away from danger.

RED ALERT

Life today tends to be at a pace never experienced by any previous generation; it feels as though we are always on 'red alert'. When the parasympathetic nervous system (also known as the peacemaker), which regulates normal function, is unable to act, the consequences range from irregular heartbeat to reproduction problems.

In this state, our muscles remain tense, our eyes keenly looking for danger. Our digestive system and other organs do not receive the blood supply they need for normal function. The heart remains beating too fast, trying to get us out of danger. Adrenalin, the hormone released in times of stress, is still running. We do not switch over to our peacemaker.

With the use of JHFM we are helping to re-educate these pathways by allowing the recipient to reconnect with a feeling of peace and calm. We are accessing the whole physical and emotional system in one treatment via the acupressure points and meridians. There is a release of energetic blockages, bringing back regular functions of the endocrine system, which regulates our hormonal balance. Those shoulders that remain tense can release and the headache from tense muscles and gritting teeth will dissolve. As we rectify the imbalances, the releasing of tense, nervous energy improves well-being, and dis-ease is replaced by calm and peace.

IN A NUTSHELL

- Japanese Holistic Face Massage has been preserved over time by the Geisha. Some of the techniques date back more than 4000 years.

- JHFM is holistic because it improves the recipient physically, mentally and emotionally.

- There is no other natural facelift treatment that utilises deep massage movements, application of acupressure and a ritual of tracing meridian points around the face and head with the fingertips.

- JHFM is a great treatment for everyone, especially the terminally ill and those suffering physical degeneration (wasting of the muscles) or mental illness.

- JHFM can be incorporated into many other massage and beauty routines.

- JHFM improves the skin's ability to renew cells, allowing regrowth, and encourages the skin's natural oils – the acid mantle (see Chapter 4).

- JHFM improves skin elasticity leaving skin soft and supple, and aids circulation, nourishing muscles and improving their tone.

- The rhythmic movement of JHFM improves the overall colour of the skin.

- JHFM encourages lymphatic flow, reducing puffiness and swelling.

- Improvement of blood supply helps repair thread veins.

- JHFM prevents blemishes occurring and improves dry mature skins.

- Massage releases tension in tired muscles by removing lactic acid.

- Massage encourages a healthy lymphatic system.

4

Skin Care

LOOKING GOOD AND MAKING OTHERS FEEL GOOD

I love looking good! I love helping others to look and feel good too. Looking good gives me confidence and is part of being good to my body. It may not be a virtue, but it's part of our world now and, as already mentioned, extremely important in Japanese culture where beauty is viewed as synonymous with longevity.

This section is devoted to understanding the structure and functions of skin and gives guidance in knowing what to look for to improve skin. The face reflects our personality and is a mirror deep into our soul. As part of our survival skills, we are born with the ability to read faces. Many people have instinctive knowledge of this and use this skill subconsciously.

SKIN DIAGNOSIS

Before you start your routine, you must check the skin's condition: is it overly oily, dry, flaky or dehydrated? Heat, wind, air conditioning, central heating, pollution and changes in temperature all have an impact on the health of skin. Many people are not aware that central heating is very drying to skin. The stress of living increasingly hectic lives can also mean there is not enough time to eat correctly and exercise. Add smoking, drinking and bad skincare and you have a range of factors that can cause skin to be old before its time.

MAIN POINTS TO CHECK

If you wish to use this routine with skincare products, it is necessary to diagnose the skin in order to decide on the type of products to use. The skin should be inspected after the facial cleanse, but you must be aware of the changes that can occur during this procedure. Changes to the skin can be the result of the particular preparation used, client anxiety or stimulation of the surface area (capillaries). The hormones may be unbalanced – during a menstrual cycle or the menopause, for example – causing the capillaries to be sensitive to internal and external influences.

The main considerations before treatments are:

- sensitivity

- surface thread veins (capillaries)

- fine lines

- skin imperfections such as blackheads (comedones), whiteheads (milia) and blemishes

- allergies (e.g. to cocoa butter which is found in many products)

- any skin complaint (e.g. eczema).

The protective layer of the skin contains fatty acids, lipid and cellular matter, which protect the skin from bacteria and external drying elements. The natural oil level can be reduced by continually washing with soap or using harsh products and as a result of exterior damage from air-borne pollutants, weather and ill health. In younger skin there is often overactive secretion of sebum from sebaceous glands, leaving skin oily due to hormonal imbalance. This can cause enlarged pores and a shiny, thick appearance due to the build-up of dead cells.

SKIN COLOUR

We are protected from the sun's rays by melanin, which is activated by the sun's rays. The more our skin is exposed to the sun, the more melanin the skin contains. Pale skin produces very little melanin, while darker skin produces a great deal more, preventing the skin from burning. Discolouration can be caused by overexposure to the sun. This will be especially noticeable on older skin. Dark patches of melanin are known as vitiligo, and partial loss of pigmentation is called chloasma.

SKIN MOISTURE

Skin that lacks moisture is referred to as dry skin, which is susceptible to premature ageing. There is a natural film that covers the skin to protect it from water evaporation. The use of moisturiser also protects the skin from water loss, which can be exacerbated in hot and cold weather, winds and centrally heated rooms.

SKIN TEMPERATURE

Environmental and body temperature has an impact on the colour and warmth of the skin. Some skin types can be instantly affected by the environment, emotional states, hormone levels or physical exertion. Dramatically increased blood circulation can restrict or flood the skin surface, the capillaries, which results in a visible change in facial appearance. In the case of those with very thin epidermis, the dilation of these capillaries as a result of additional blood flow to the face will be noticeable and the face will appear red or flushed.

OIL ACID/ALKALINE LEVELS – ACID MANTLE

The pH level of facial skin is between 5 and 5.6, resulting in an acid reaction. The neutral pH balance is 7. The acid balance is composed of oil (sebum), sweat and the process of shedding skin cells (keratinisation), and is called the 'acid mantle'. It protects the skin from invasion from bacteria, other micro-organisms and pollution, and prevents the evaporation of the skin's moisture content.

When you use harsh products, they will have a drying effect, leaving the skin stretched and taut, especially on dry and sensitive types, and aggravating the condition of the skin. These harsh products, together with pollutants, destroy the acid mantle, leaving the skin defenceless for a period of time until it is able to reform.

SKIN TYPES

Greasy skin

Skin appears shiny with evidence of excessive oily secretions, especially around the nose, forehead and chin. Greasy skin is usually coarse with open pores and is prone to blemishes. This condition is due to overactive functioning of the sebaceous glands (see the image on page 35). An overzealous facial routine can aggravate the condition because it can remove the acid mantle. Neglecting to care for the skin will lead to a steady build-up of dead cells, leaving the skin vulnerable to germs and environmental damage.

Combination skin

This type of skin is identified by an oily middle section of the face, forehead, nose and chin areas, which appear greasy, while the sides of the face are drier. Ideally, you should treat both sections separately. Treatment will be necessary for the open pores round the nose, chin and forehead, and the possible formation of blackheads.

Normal skin

Normal skin has a lovely glow, is matt, not too oily, too dry or too moist. When wiped with a facial tissue, there should be no evidence of moisture. It is soft and supple to touch and will benefit from the use of natural products in order to keep it healthy, attractive and young-looking.

Dry skin

This type of skin appears fine, taut, parched, transparent and often flaky. There is a tendency towards transparency, especially in older skins. Very dry skin takes on a crepey aspect and ages much more quickly than normal or greasy skin. Fine lines often appear around the eyes at an early age. There is an absence of open pores and a tendency towards sensitivity, with the surface often lined and wrinkled. There is a lack of protective sebum, so this skin reacts quickly to extreme weather conditions, resulting in chapped and rough skin.

Dehydrated

The skin appearance is crepey with dilated capillaries and dry scaly areas. There are open, relaxed pores, especially around the cheeks, under the nose and in the chin area, and fine lines can be seen around the eyes and mouth. There is a tendency for older skins to become dehydrated where there is a gradual deterioration in the metabolism and circulation, preventing renewal of healthy skin tissue, due to ill health or inadequate diet. Younger skins, even if naturally oily, can become dehydrated with dry, scaly patches.

BE GOOD TO YOUR SKIN

Natural products are recommended to enhance and cleanse effectively without irritation or excessive manipulation (roughness), especially oily types, which are easily stimulated (acne rosacea), to avoid causing further damage.

UNDERSTANDING SKIN PRODUCTS – BENEFITS AND USES
Cleansers

There are many reasons for cleansing: dust from the atmosphere, perspiration, oily patches and stale makeup on the surface of the skin. A good cleanser contains nutrients and, when massaged into the skin, will be easily absorbed, improving the health and condition of the skin. It is formulated to dissolve the oils, waxes and pigments in cosmetics without breaking down the skin's defence barrier (acid mantle). Cleansers have a vital effect on the function of the skin, its tendency to age, its appearance and protection from blemishes and pollutants.

Toners

Many people neglect using a toner and will regret this when they are older. A toner stimulates the pores to contract, thereby maintaining a lovely clear, smooth complexion. Open pores can be a sign of excessive sebum production. The application of a toner helps to remove excess oil and closes the pores to protect invasion from bacteria and micro-organisms. Toners protect against infections, blemishes, boils, blackheads and whiteheads, and have a cooling and calming effect. Most household brands of cosmetics contain alcohol, which means that they dry out the skin and tend to have a high acid level which disrupts or even destroys the acid mantle on the face. Look for brands that are organic or that only use natural ingredients. These tend not to include alcohol and will include ingredients that nourish the skin. They are surprisingly cheaper than many household brands. A toner should be used after cleansing and after exfoliation. Using a toner will refine the pores as they relax after gentle massage, remove excess cleanser and cool the face ready for moisturising.

Moisturisers

What would we do without our moisturiser? Vital for keeping skin looking young regardless of age, it must be used daily. Moisturisers help protect the skin from loss of moisture. Each cell in our body is roughly 70 per cent water. Without an adequate intake of water, skin cells become dehydrated and die. The dead cells clog the skin, creating a barrier between healthy cells and causing the skin to become irritated, dull and unsightly. Even naturally oily skin can have dry patches that will crack, giving the appearance of an uneven surface. These are perfect conditions for the incubation of germs, causing blemishes and boils, and a formation of dust and dirt in pores.

Moisturisers vary and are adapted to different skin types. They contain water and oils that naturally nourish and protect, including protection from UVA and UVB rays. Many plant oils have natural ingredients that protect and will not dry out the skin.

An efficient moisturiser keeps skin soft and supple regardless of skin type; the oilier the skin, the more water used within the moisturiser. Richer moisturisers contain a higher proportion of oil to water. All form a protective barrier to keep natural protective oils in. The higher the water content, the higher the evaporation rate.

Exfoliants

If you want to maintain beautiful skin and ensure the entire product range you are using is working to its optimum, it is important to exfoliate. Exfoliate! Whatever your age, you should be looking after your skin. Over time, cellular matter will make your skin dull, lifeless and prone to infection, promoting the ageing process. Summer sun will stimulate the skin's metabolism, which will then slow down in the winter. There is also a quicker build-up of cellular matter when you have naturally oily or younger skin. This means it is necessary to exfoliate frequently – for example, once or twice a week. For more mature skin, exfoliation once a week or every two weeks is fine. Exfoliates should not contain harsh ingredients as these only aggravate the skin and may cause damage to all skin types. There is a vast range now available. Look for soft grains, not harsh or gritty products. These are the easiest to use; however, the 'rub-off' types are more efficient, if a little fiddly. The trick is not to *scrub* the skin but to use gentle, short sliding movements, with the ring finger working into the skin. Then rinse off.

Face masks

Masks are a vital part of anyone's facial routine, allowing for intensive care of problem areas, no matter what the skin type. Masks ensure that the skin is deep-cleansed, revitalised and nourished, the pores refined and the outer skin texture evened.

Types of face masks

- Setting masks contain natural clays. They bring impurities to the surface. They can either calm or stimulate.

- Non-setting masks contain natural ingredients and affect the surface moisture of the skin.

- Specialised masks can be peel-off gels or non-setting and are designed to tackle problem skins, including oily or mature skin. They can be made from natural ingredients or chemicals.

Classification of masks

- Stimulating – to encourage circulation on sallow skin.

- Emollient – to clear inflamed skin and soften and nourish dry skin.

- Astringent – for coarse, oily skin.

- Demulcent – soothing for inflamed skin.

- Tonic – to improve the tone of the skin.

Eye moisturiser

This is an important part of a beauty routine regardless of skin type and regardless of age. The delicate area around the eyes needs special care in order to prevent puffy eyes, dark circles and fine lines. Moisturisers should never be applied here; the ingredients are too harsh and will encourage puffiness under the eyes and may cause inflammation. There are different formulas available, usually containing herbs and plant oils, and they come in creams, balms or gels. Gels are more soothing for problem delicate skin. Creams are designed mainly to prevent fine lines. All will encourage circulation and nourish the skin.

Lip moisturiser

To protect from the sun's rays and nourish dry lips, use a good lip moisturiser. Again, these have different functions: some will plump the lips, while others protect from harsh conditions such as wind and cold. This area of the skin is thin and vulnerable and should not be overlooked in a beauty routine.

Never use a mineral oil, such as paraffin oil, which goes through various stages of chemical processing to become an oil or ointment. Mineral oils tend to create a barrier on the skin and act as an occlusive, preventing water loss. Mineral oils cannot easily be washed off and therefore cause the pores to become clogged with particles. You may feel initially that they soften your lips; however, over time the lips become dry and scaly, preventing nutrients from penetrating the lips. Natural lip moisturisers are designed to protect and nourish rather than block.

IN A NUTSHELL

- Looking good on the outside makes you feel good inside.

- Recognise skin type – oily, combination, dry or dehydrated – and use the correct skin products.

- Check for broken capillaries and skin sensitivity to heat.

- The skin's natural protective layer – the acid mantle – needs to be maintained through the correct cleansing and moisturising regime.

- Using natural products will enhance your skin in the long term, preventing problems occurring.

- Cleansers remove impurities as well as makeup.

- Toners prevent large unsightly pores by clearing dirt and oils, and refining the pores.

- Moisturisers nourish and protect the skin from damage.

- Eye moisturisers prevent puffiness, dark circles and fine lines.

- Lip moisturisers give protection from harsh weather conditions and plump the lips, adding to their beauty.

5

What is Japanese Holistic Face Massage?

I have explained about the differences between Western and Eastern culture and attitude towards health, and how massage has always been a big part of the Japanese way of life. The Japanese Holistic Face Massage (JHFM) sequence of movements is based on 4000 years of knowledge, rooted in a holistic approach to health and well-being. The JHFM routine delivers everything a Western facial does and then goes further by invigorating the recipient's health and enhancing their beauty. The following is a brief summary of the facial massage.

WHO WILL BENEFIT?

Japanese Holistic Face Massage is wonderfully therapeutic and can be enjoyed by anyone who receives it as a treatment. Due to its completely holistic nature, I believe it can be particularly beneficial to a range of individuals and circumstances, and here's why. JHFM has the ability to calm the mind under traumatic circumstances and is a particularly good treatment for the terminally ill. At times we need to feel reassurance and have a sense of inner peace. JHFM helps to lift a patient's mood and stimulate lost appetite. In circumstances where there is physical degeneration such as muscle atrophy, the release of blocked negative energy can stimulate regeneration on a neurological and muscular level.

It is a perfect addition to the toolkit of healthcare professionals, especially those working in hospices, nursing homes and hospitals. It can work nicely alongside Western medicine by allowing those who are very ill to find the strength to move forward in their recovery or, conversely, the strength to face their oncoming death with grace and peace.

This massage has amazing results for those who are caring for relatives at home. Any adult or child with chronic disorders, disability or emotional frailty will benefit greatly from this treatment. The energetic connection between the practitioner and recipient plays an important part in the healing process as it is one of the purest expressions of love combined with physical touch. Healing on the emotional level helps to improve the recipient's response to conventional medicine.

ADAPTATION OF THE MOVEMENTS

Although the massage should ideally be done using a massage bed, the movements can also be adapted for use while the recipient is sitting in a chair or wheelchair. Although not ideal, as long as the therapist is standing above the patient's head and can see the recipient's face and reach their shoulders, it is possible to give the massage.

For therapists working in hospitals, a hospital bed is very suitable as the bed head can be lowered, much like a massage bed, while the therapist sits at the head to perform the routine.

PERFECT AS A NEW TREATMENT

Holistic therapists who want to include a unique treatment that will benefit their clients physiologically and psychologically will find JHFM a great addition to the treatment options they can offer. It is a perfect treatment to calm and release anxiety or tension. I also integrate this treatment with other therapies such as reflexology, reiki, aromatherapy and deep tissue back massage. I find it significantly improves a client's response to the other treatments due to the relaxed state and the release of blocked Ki. Part one of JHFM can also be used separately – for example, beauty therapists can use this part as a beauty treatment. Part one can also be incorporated into other massage routines.

NO OTHER NATURAL FACELIFT LIKE JHFM

There is no other natural facelift routine that incorporates all these deep massage movements, the application of acupressure and ritual of tracing the points of meridians around the face and head with the fingertips. The process of tracing the meridians regulates the flow of Ki from the lowest number acupressure point to the highest. Beginning at the large bowel and continuing on to Ren Mai (see massage routine below) completes the natural energy loop. The Ki energy connection on all levels gives the recipients extra release. Other routines will regulate acupressure points but they do not consider directional flow which ultimately gives a more powerful result each time.

A WORD ABOUT IMAGINATION

Without imagination we cannot open our minds to ideas and subjects that are unfamiliar. It is the precursor of being a more spiritual being. When we slow down our breathing, we are allowing the constant chatter to subside. We open ourselves to new sensations and learn new skills. Things that do not come as second nature are suddenly revealed to us, enabling us to raise our own vibration.

SPIRITUAL CONNECTION – A THREE-WAY CONNECTION

When you give this massage with the intention of helping another person, you are setting up a three-way energetic connection and no effort on your part is required. Just relax and enjoy the experience. 'Thoughts' are a type of energy, and when a thought is good and positive, the vibration of the thinker is raised. This vibration then connects with the heavens (universe or source). Positioning yourself above the person's head makes this connection easier to attain. Working with energy does not mean you need to know about spirituality; you just have to have an appreciation of its existence.

If you are in a salon environment or do not feel confident, the following simple method is a practical alternative to setting the connection:

- Sit with a straight back at the recipient's head.

- Rest your hands on the top of the arms (deltoids) and take 20 seconds for your breathing to settle.

- Move your hands to the centre of the chest, just below the clavicle, to begin.

- Setting the mood allows you both to relax.

OPTIONAL OPENING MOVEMENTS

- When you have positioned yourself, lay your hands down on the upper part of the chest, close to the collar bone (clavicle), with your fingertips facing.

- Breathe gently through your nose until your breathing has settled (this should take about 10–20 seconds). Then breathe out and imagine the air you breathed out (energy) going through the recipient's body and out through their feet.

- Next, ask the recipient to breathe in and, as they do so, you breathe in simultaneously, adding a slight pressure on the upper chest in rhythm to the expansion of the chest. Once again, imagine the breath coming, this time from above your head, down through you and down through the recipient's body and out through their feet.

- If you wish, you can actively engage the recipient by asking them to breathe in through their nose and out through their mouth. Ask them to imagine the breath going down through to their abdomen, hips, thighs, legs and out through their feet on the out breath.

- These simple actions set the mood for the massage, allowing you also to settle and begin. This is an optional move and may not suit everyone.

Your hands are now in the perfect position to start this unique massage. However, before you start, you really need to understand how to access the acupressure points. I therefore suggest you read the next section carefully.

ENERGETIC ALLIANCE

Once you have completed the first section of the massage, it is time to go deeper, using the acupressure routine. This is a truly outstanding treatment which benefits the giver as well as the recipient. Bringing this pure healing energy to your conscious mind enhances the flow of pure healing energy where it is needed most. This is a wonderful massage to give as well as receive.

- The breath is an essential part of your connection to the acupressure points. Be aware as you breathe in and out through the nose. Feel the breath coming up, from your abdomen, expanding across from your heart and down your arms through to your middle or ring fingers as your fingers rest on the points. Relax and let this happen.

- As the connection grows, bring into your awareness energy coming down from your head to your heart as you breathe in, expanding out from the heart.

- This should be a steady flow, not rigid. Allow your shoulders to relax, letting your breath flow in unison with the recipient's, breathing in through your nose and out through your nose, up through the abdomen and down from your head, meeting at the heart and expanding down to your fingertips.

- It will feel like a meditation. This means you are completely in the moment, your awareness on all sensations around you.

- You are now connected to heaven and earth, balancing energy and helping the recipient to release anxiety, stress and tension to bring in healing, a sense of calm and peace of mind.

- When a rapport in breathing is established, start to concentrate on the differences between the points, letting your gaze become softer, your breath even and expansive.

Of course, all of the above will become easier with practice. In all, it should only take 30–45 seconds to establish the connection, and when you are proficient, it will easily become part of your practice. The trick is to relax and let go, rather than control. A note of caution: do not expect to keep the connection throughout. It takes much concentration and practice to achieve, but it will come in time. Your mind will naturally wander and that is normal. Just bring your mind back to your breath.

PRACTISE ON YOURSELF

The best way to understand the energy section of this routine is to practice first on yourself. Do not be in a hurry to give to others until you master the key parts, especially awareness of the subtle differences within Ki energy. The more you practise, the more you will develop your skills of distinguishing one point from the other. You will also personally feel the benefits. When you are confident, it is time to try your skills on family and friends. When you start to practise on others, you will be amazed at their reactions.

Remember, it is a three-way connection between you, the soft, nurturing aspect of the earth and the empowering knowledge of the universe. Establishing this three-way connection will bring harmony and balance.

Connecting and listening to the energetic points is like being at a concert. As the members of the orchestra tune their instruments, a myriad of sounds vibrates through the air. Then, suddenly, a sweet sound of harmony prevails and you are swept away with the resonance and perfection of the moment.

A light gentle pressure allows you to feel the differences, bilaterally. As awareness grows, increase the pressure slightly, in a circular motion, out towards the ears. Never apply strong pressure. Feel the differences one side to the other. Imagine the points as cups that gently open, are stimulated and finally close again. The response under your fingers may be soft or feel empty as if that pool is stagnant. This means there is an excess of Yin. If the point being pressed feels firm, it means there is excess Yang. These points are intrinsically linked to the aspect of the meridians you are working. Think of those pools of emotion: is there an overreaction or is it dark and empty?

FEELING CHANNELS POINT TO POINT

The next step is to trace the meridian through the energetic symmetric loop, as Ki energy passes through the body. There is a strict order, starting with the lowest number acupressure point and progressing to the highest. Simultaneously sweep through each meridian with your fingertips.

A STREAM OF VIBRANT WATER

As you gently trace the meridian points, think of a vibrant, energised stream of clear water rushing through the channels. Upon meeting an obstacle, imagine gently releasing the stream so it can continue its onward, fluid journey. Remember that each organ has a partner, together with the two single extraordinary vessels. You are connecting to the whole energetic system, encouraging a balancing flow of energy, completing the loop and the directional flow, creating harmony and resonance.

PROPERTIES OF THE INDIVIDUAL POINT

Each acupressure point has individual emotional or physical attributes. Acupressure points are located close to sensory and motor nerves, to individual muscles or muscle groups. When these are massaged, they offer a quick response to ailments such as sinusitis, headache, migraine or neck and shoulder pain. Ki energy relieves pain locally, while having a ripple effect on the whole body systems.

COMPLETE THE MASSAGE

At the end of the massage, on your last out breath, imagine the breath going through the recipient's body and out through their feet to the ground. You can also do the same action on yourself; then simply wash your hands, as you do so washing off any negativity you may have picked up energetically. Alternatively, allow your hands to slide down gently over the arms and the legs towards the feet, taking all the energy back to earth. This also helps to ground the recipient.

IN A NUTSHELL

- Initially, practise on yourself to allow you to feel differences from one side of the head and face to the other.

- Never apply strong pressure.

- Use your creativity and imagination to learn the differences in the energy from point to point.

- One way is to imagine that the meridians are channels of vibrant water, clearing all obstacles (impurities) in their path.

- Maintain steady, relaxed breathing throughout the routine.

- Focus in order to prevent constant mind chatter.

- The optional movement will not suit everyone.

- Establishing a three-way connection between you, the recipient and the universal life source is key to the routine.

- Remember to ground the recipient and yourself after treatment.

Benefits of JHFM

- Promotes healing by accessing all body organs via meridians and pressure points.

- Releases toxins in skin tissue and throughout the body back into the lymph.

- Lymphatic drainage aids cell renewal and reduces puffiness to the face, neck and shoulders, while also improving the flow of body fluid throughout the body.

- Stimulates muscle tone.

- Targets specific disorders by releasing blocked Ki.

- Balances deficient and stagnating Ki energy and improves directional flow, thereby rebalancing the whole body emotionally and spiritually.

- Helps realign chakras.

- Produces a wonderful sense of well-being, confidence, vitality and a more positive outlook.

6

Getting Started

It is important to know if there are any reasons why this massage cannot take place. If, for example, you are a volunteer in a nursing home, hospice or hospital, permission from the nursing staff, family doctor or registrar assigned to the patient must be given.

The massage therapist will need to be aware of any contraindications and have a full history of the client. As a carer, you will already be aware of any reason not to give this massage; however, it is always best to seek advice from the recipient's doctor or other disciplines involved in their care. Age is not a concern as all ages respond well and benefit from this treatment.

CONTRAINDICATIONS

Anybody wishing to undertake this massage must be aware of the following:

- allergies to cosmetics and foodstuffs

- fever

- recent surgery, dental work or injury (in the last six weeks)

- acne or rosacea

- any inflammatory skin condition which appears on the face, neck or shoulders

- a severe cold or contagious illness

- cuts or open sores.

AFTERCARE

Ensure that the recipient has water, preferably at room temperature in order not to overstimulate the digestive system. Encourage them to drink at least one glass of water following treatment. This will improve the rate of the removal of toxins and waste out of the body after treatment.

BEFORE YOU BEGIN

Things to take into consideration:

- The room should be comfortable and well-ventilated. There must be privacy to ensure the recipient can remain relaxed and not be distracted by noise or people.

- Ensure that the person is warm, with towels or blankets ready to cover the shoulders. Extra covers are useful for the feet, as our body temperature drops when we relax.

- If you carry out the massage while seated, make sure you have positioned yourself correctly. You must be able to reach the recipient easily without invading their space.

- Always keep your back straight, your shoulders and wrists relaxed. Adjust your chair or use cushions to ensure you are at the correct height.

- It is not advisable to stand while giving this massage unless the recipient is in a chair or wheelchair for their comfort.

Everyone is different and it is about intuitively knowing the person you are massaging. The pressure can vary from person to person, especially the opening movements that concentrate on the neck and shoulders. Remain aware of any small response to your touch. Remember to warm the muscles well. This will help loosen tired muscles, making the rotation of the head easier and the recipient more relaxed.

FACIAL CLEANSE ROUTINE

It is essential to properly clean traces of makeup, dirt and impurities before you start a facial routine. The cleanse routine below will guide you through the steps, and diagrams are included on the pages that follow.

- Stroke across the forehead.

- Seven strokes across the neck, ending with the left hand.

- Four and a half strokes along the jaw.

- Stroke the outer side of cheeks and jaw to the centre cheek, then to the eyes and finally up the centre towards the corner of the eyes.

- Thumb kneading to the chin.

- Ring finger up the laughter lines, along the top of the lip, around nostrils six times.

- Stroking movements up the side of the nose with the index and middle finger.

- Stroking movements over the procerus muscle, using the ring fingers only, six times.

- Forehead stroking six times.

- Pressure at the temples to finish.

The full luxury facial

The following is a basic guide to giving a full luxury facial. This routine is used by many beauty therapists and is included as additional information for those who want to know how to do a full facial but don't have a beauty therapy background.

- Cleanse face twice with natural skin care products to suit skin type.

- Tone.

- Exfoliate to remove dead cells.

- Tone again.

- Use massage oil that complements the massage and treatment, paying attention to any meridians that you feel need extra attention.

- Do not remove oil – apply a mask on top of it, and leave for about 5–10 minutes.

- Tone.

- Apply eye moisturiser, lip moisture and face moisturiser.

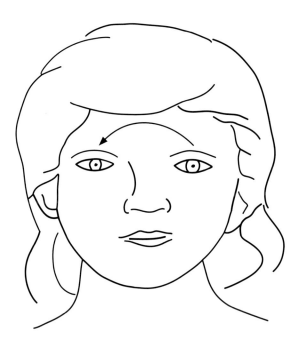

1. STROKE ACROSS THE FOREHEAD

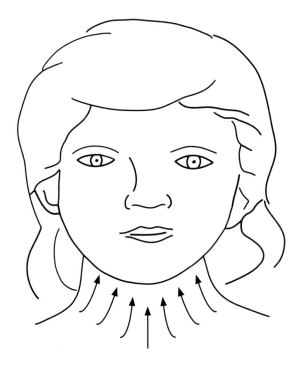

2. SEVEN STROKES UP THE NECK, ENDING WITH THE LEFT HAND

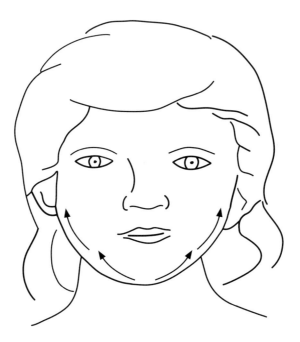

3. FOUR AND A HALF STROKES ALONG THE JAW

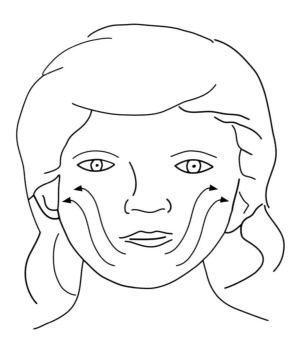

4. EFFLEURAGE (STROKING) UP THE CENTRE TOWARDS
THE TEMPLES, USING THE WHOLE HAND

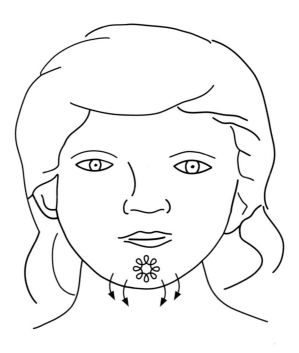

5. THUMB KNEADING THE CHIN AREA

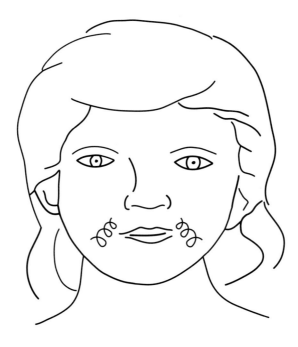

6. USING THE RING FINGERS, CIRCULAR MOVEMENTS UP THE
LAUGHTER LINES, ALONG THE TOP LIP AND AROUND THE NOSTRILS

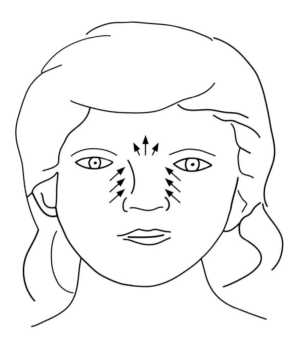

7. STROKING THE SIDE OF THE NOSE, USING THE INDEX
AND MIDDLE FINGERS, LEFT SIDE THEN RIGHT, THEN OVER
THE PROCERUS MUSCLE USING THE RING FINGER

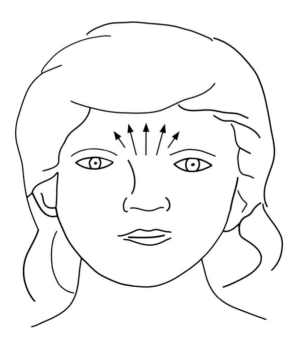

8. FOREHEAD STROKING, FINISHING WITH
LIGHT PRESSURE AT THE TEMPLES

Now that you have a thorough background and history of this fantastic treatment, the following are short introductions to each segment. Remember, this is a modular treatment, meaning you can use segments of it in conjunction with other routines. The segments you use will depend on how you choose to adapt it.

OPTIONAL CLEANSE ROUTINE

As with any other facial, there is an optional basic cleanse/tone routine to remove dirt and makeup (see page 62). This is also an opportunity to diagnose the condition of the skin and what natural skincare products would be best to use for the individual.

OPTIONAL OPENING MOVEMENTS

First, there are the optional opening movements (see page 54) setting the mood for the whole massage, which will help you and your client to remain relaxed throughout. The opening movements can either be carried out before or after the optional cleanse.

Each movement within the segments should be repeated 3–4 times, unless instructed otherwise.

PART ONE: OPENING MOVEMENTS
Neck and shoulder movements 1–6

These are mainly effleurage movements and some manipulation, relaxing and warming the muscle groups. While also giving a slight stretch to the neck, this action releases tension. There are small rotations of the head, to a 45-degree angle, further loosening neck muscles. Other movements follow the contours of the shoulders to the neck, adding slight lifts to achieve release and relaxation. Gentle percussion to the neck helps to stimulate circulation and lymphatic flow. Other movements bring the energy up from the neck and shoulders towards the face. Nutrients are stimulated and encouraged to flood the muscle and the dermis, releasing lactic acid and toxins back to the lymphatic vessels.

If you are a massage professional, you may find that many of the movements do not follow the usual massage routine. Remember that this is a set of traditional movements used in amna (traditional Japanese massage). Many of the movements are used to treat injuries and over time have been integrated into Japanese Holistic Face Massage.

Facial massage movements 7–22

This section combines effleurage, petrissage and tapotement to achieve suppleness of the skin and muscles. It brings nutrients deep into the skin and connective tissue, as well as the muscle tissue. Toxins are released via the lymphatic system. This series of movements can, at times, be more rigorous than a normal facial, although not overly aggressive. There is lifting of facial muscle, encouraging tired muscles to release, across the mandible (jaw), mentalis (chin), zygomatic (cheeks) and occipitofrontalis (forehead) muscles. The movements should never be uncomfortable to the recipient.

PART TWO: MERIDIAN MOVEMENTS 23–31

Allow yourself plenty of time to complete this section as the experience of giving as well as receiving is totally relaxing. Having already ensured the establishment of the three-way connection between yourself, the recipient and the universal life force, now just relax your shoulders and wrists and concentrate on bringing in positive energy and releasing the negative. The movements in this section will allow healing to take place on all levels. Using your middle or ring fingers, remember to perform bilaterally so you can feel the difference between one side and the other. Start at the lowest number acupressure point (tsubo) and do not forget to trace each individual meridian after you have mapped out the points. If you forget, then go back and trace before going on to the next series of points.

PART THREE: FINAL MOVEMENTS 32–36

This section focuses on encouraging the venous return. Light massage, working superficially on the skin, returns cell debris, deoxygenated blood and toxins back into the lymph, to be carried away from the face and out of the body. This starts the healing process and renewal of cells, enhances skin colour, gives a smooth complexion, releases tiredness and diminishes fine lines. If you are using these movements as part of a facial routine, you can now apply the mask, and continue with the full luxury facial (page 63).

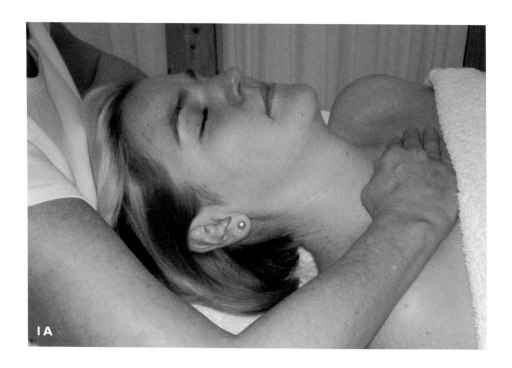

IA

PART ONE: OPENING MOVEMENTS
Neck and shoulder movements 1–6

Apply oil liberally over shoulders, neck and face using effleurage movements.

1 Opening movement: bring both hands to the centre of the chest, resting under the clavicle (collar bone). Take a deep breath and release. Slide both hands over the deltoid muscle (head of the arm bone), turn the wrist, slide along top of shoulders and grasp the neck at the base of the skull (occipital) with cupped hands, giving a lift at the same time and maintaining support.

1a Release the right hand and place flat on to the clavicle. Slide the right hand across to the deltoid and push down.

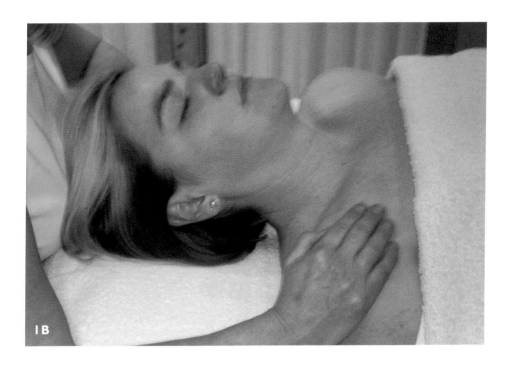

1b Turn the wrist, slide under the shoulder (scapula) and push up.

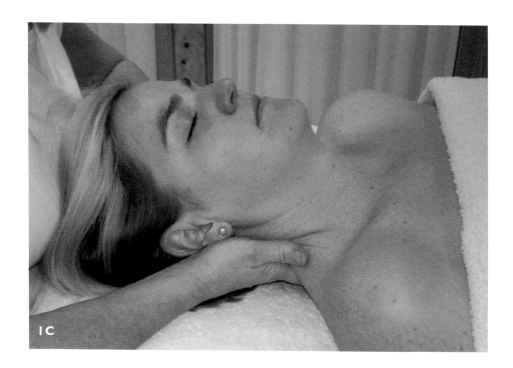

1c Maintaining pressure and, moving towards the seventh vertebra, run the fingers beside the vertebra, maintaining pressure until you meet resistance (base of the occipital). Then release pressure. Repeat on the other side.

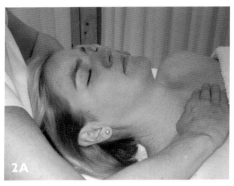
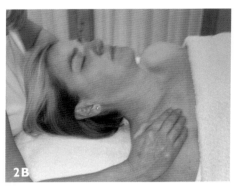
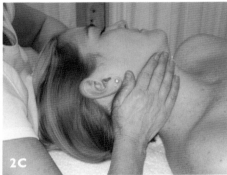

2 Place the hand just below the clavicle. Sweep around the top of the shoulder, following the contours of the neck with a flat hand to the jaw. Turn the head to a 45-degree angle to access the neck. Turn the head back to the centre. Repeat on the other side.

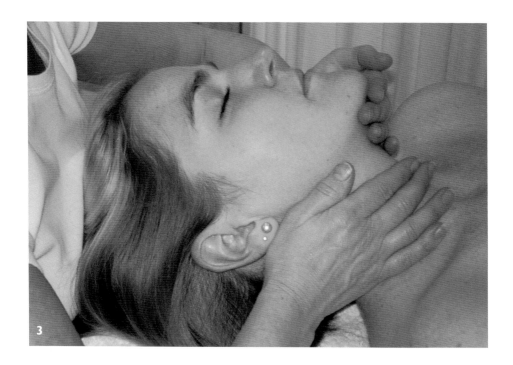

3 Use effleurage movements along the neck for 20 seconds, avoiding pressure on the oesophagus.

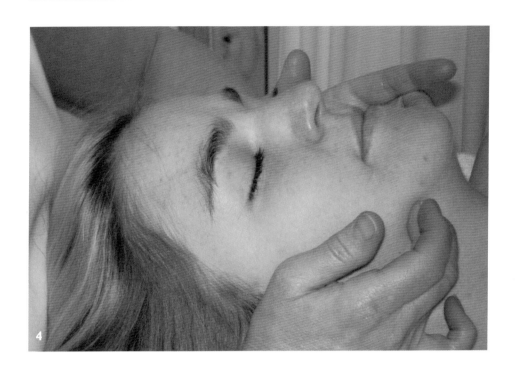

4 Using index fingers only, stroke under the chin to stimulate lymphatic flow and improve the appearance around the chin.

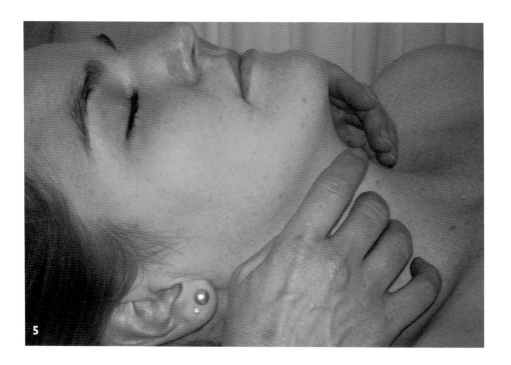

5 Apply light percussion under the chin and neck for 20 seconds. This will help to improve the chin area and stimulate blood flow to the neck tissues.

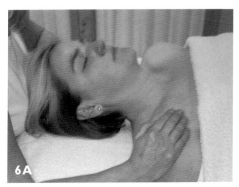
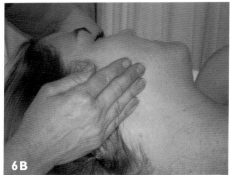

6 Turn the head to a 45-degree angle again as you sweep from the deltoid following the contour of the neck to just below the ear, using a firm effleurage movement with the whole hand. Repeat on the other side. Return the head to the centre.

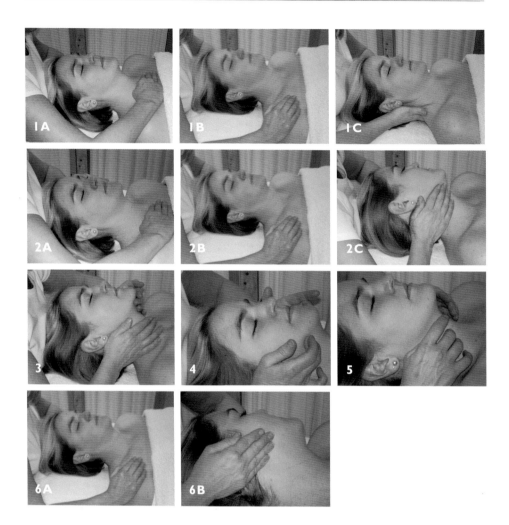

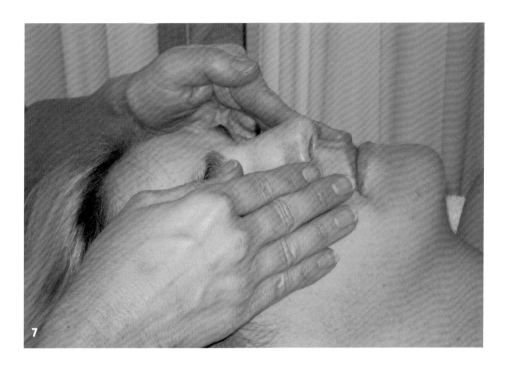

Facial massage movements 7–22

7 Using both hands, apply effleurage movements to the side of the face – first to the temple, then the outer corner of the eye, the middle of the eye and over the entire area. This increases circulation to the cheek and eye area.

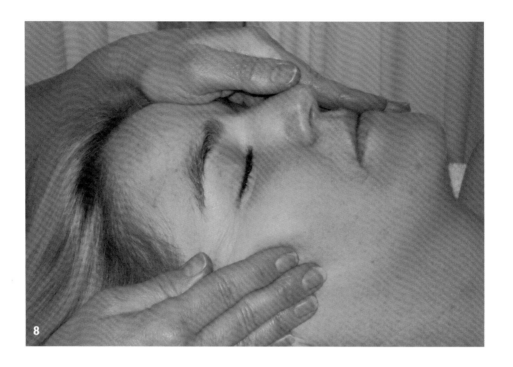

8 Place the left hand over the left side of the face with the heel of the hand on the eyebrow ridge. Again, use effleurage on the opposite cheek. This action will increase circulation, warming and relaxing the facial tissue. Repeat on the other side.

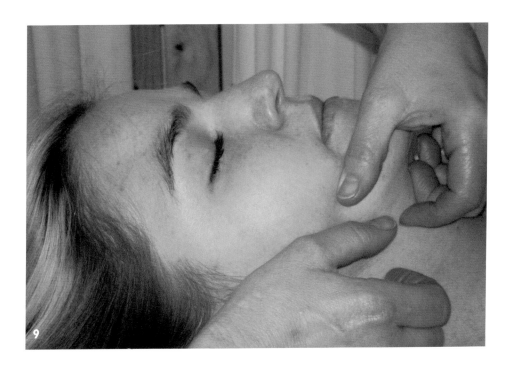

9 Flip-stroke the jawbone, using the thumbs only. Do not rest your hands on the oesophagus and avoid any pressure to the throat. This movement will stimulate facial tissue along the jaw line. Increase the pressure by changing to small circular movements, lifting the skin tissue away from the jaw, in order to release tension in the muscles.

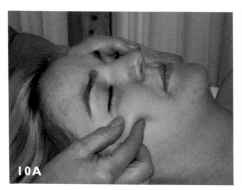 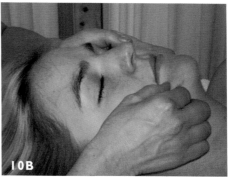

10 Gently supporting the opposite side of the head, use the thumb and index finger to lift the muscle tissue, first under the upper cheek, avoiding the eye area, and then along the chin, using the right hand for the right side and the left hand for the left side. This movement improves the action of the facial muscles, allowing nutrients in, and stimulates while releasing tension. Repeat on the other side.

Repeat the movements, lifting the muscle tissue on both cheeks simultaneously and finally across the chin.

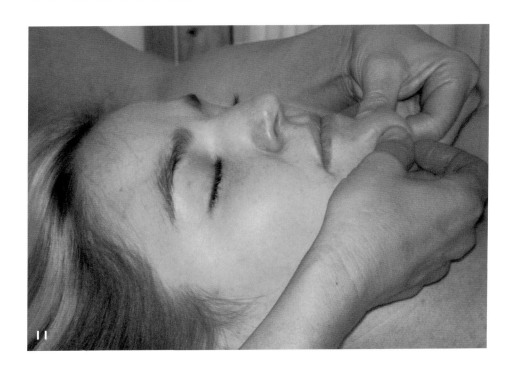

11 Knead the chin with the thumbs only for 20 seconds. This is a strong movement, lifting the muscle away from the bone. While also relaxing the chin, this increases circulation and aids the correct function of the muscles attached to the chin.

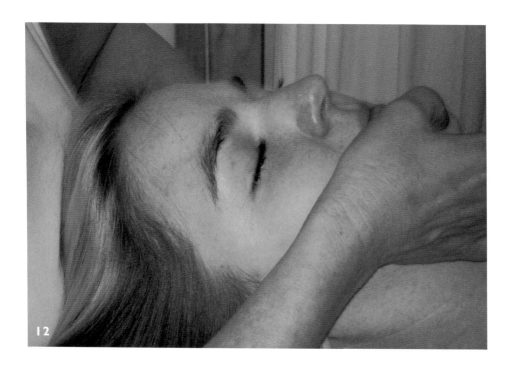

12 Rest the thumb on the centre of the chin. Inhale and breathe out gently. Pause for about 20 seconds. Apply pressure using small circular movements with the thumb at the centre of the chin. Apply pressure first and then rotate. The action should come from the shoulder rather than just the hand. This action gets deep into the muscle to release tension and aid fatigue.

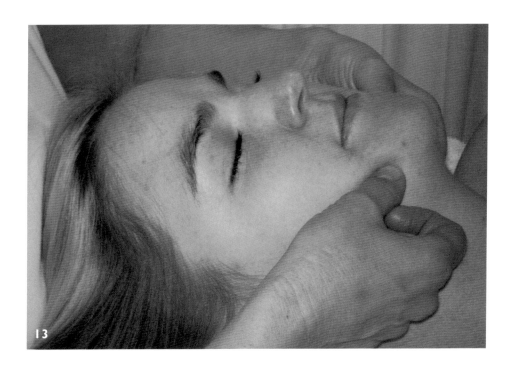

13 Using thumb pressure, repeat three times along the jaw line. This movement reduces tension along the jaw, improves appearance and helps to maintain normal function of the muscles around the jaw line. It also releases muscle fatigue.

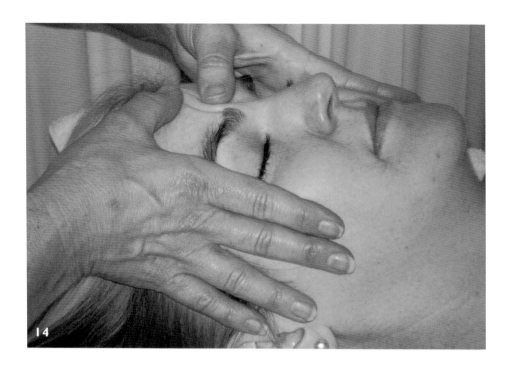

14 Apply kneading to the forehead. As you do these movements, push the centre skin gently up. This movement increases circulation, improves appearance and prevents fine lines on the forehead.

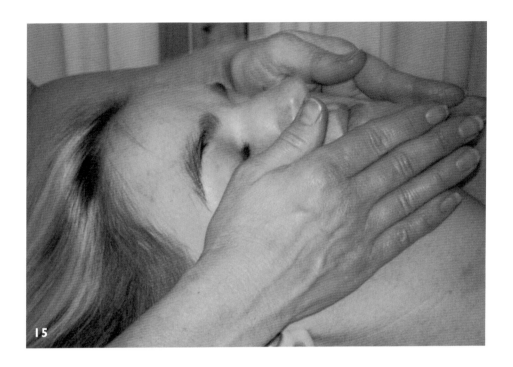

15 Using effleurage prayer movements starting at the forehead, slide down to the cheeks, coming off at the jaw. This movement clears away toxins from the lymphatic vessels located in the face.

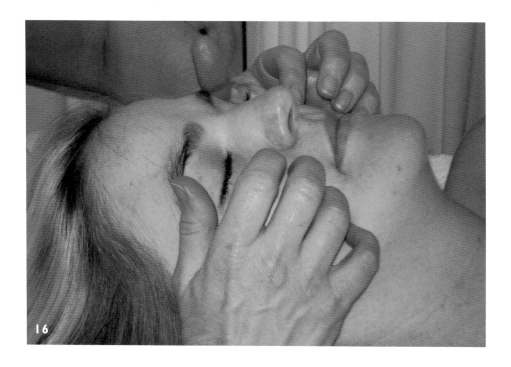

16 Using four fingers, apply light percussion on the face for 20 seconds. Gently tap the cheeks loosely with the flattened fingers, not allowing nails to touch. This movement encourages the flow of blood circulation and stimulates vascular response.

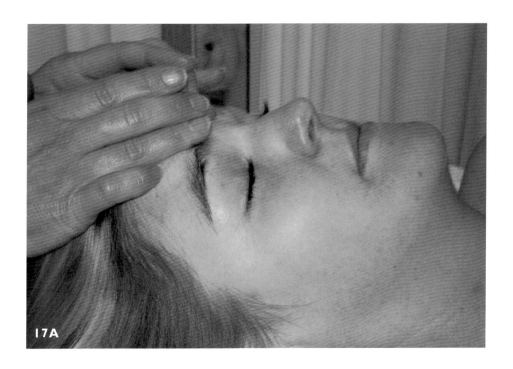

17 Finger stroking on the side of the nose must be carried out in order a, b, c and d, using the index or ring fingers. Then repeat. This movement aids the removal of dirt and oil.

17a Slide down from the nose to the corner of the mouth.

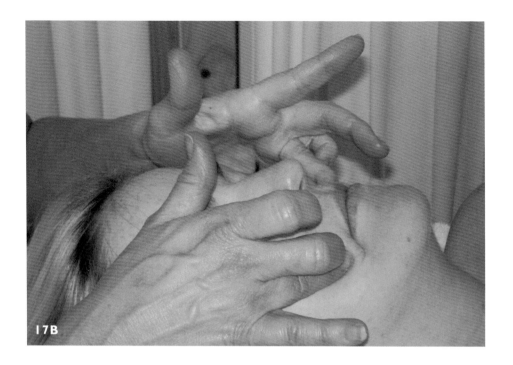

17b Slide back up from the mouth, around the nostrils.

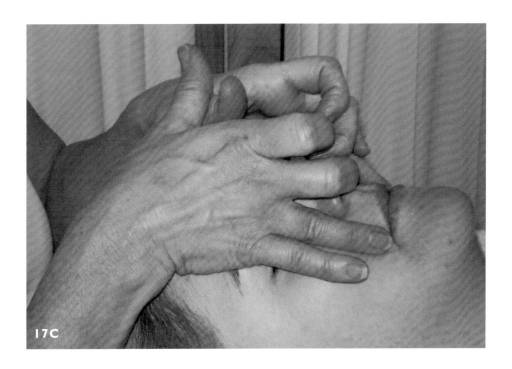

17c   Slide down from the nose to the corner of the mouth.

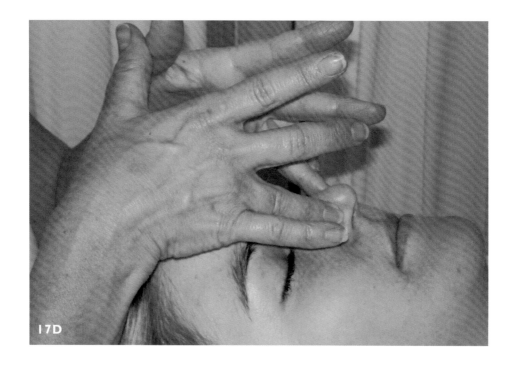

17d Slide around the nostrils and repeat the movement.

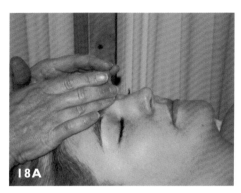
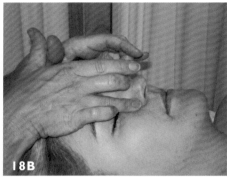

18 Slide down from the bridge of the nose to the septum. Circle around the nostrils and around the outside of the nose. Slide up to the bridge of the nose and repeat. This movement increases circulation and will open the sinuses, as well as helping with the removal of oil and grease.

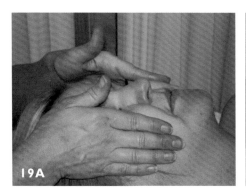
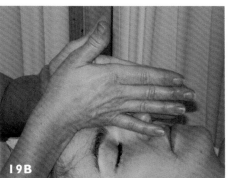

19 Smooth effleurage movements with flat hands from the forehead to the temples, over the cheek, up to the tip of the nose and off, with both hands finishing together. This effleurage prayer movement drains lymph from the forehead, while also increasing circulation to the very tip of the nose.

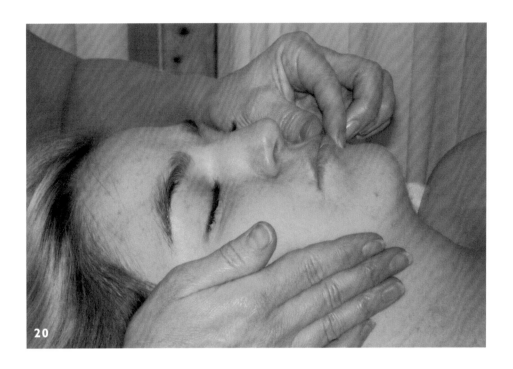

20 Lift the lips, using the thumbs and index fingers only, bringing them together. This movement improves the delicate skin of the lips.

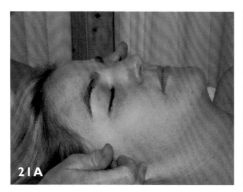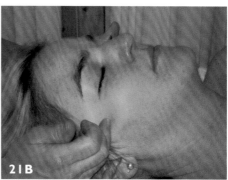

21 Using the ring or index finger in front of the ear, start midway from the corner of the eye and the top of the ear (temple area) and stroke to the top of the ear. Draw a second line perpendicular to the first and in line with the mid-ear. Repeat the movement perpendicular to the bottom of the ear. Then slide the finger up from the finishing point to the beginning with a slight lift. This movement improves the appearance of the side of the face and gives a slight lift to the facial tissue in this area. Repeat on each side.

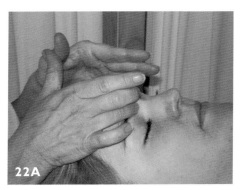 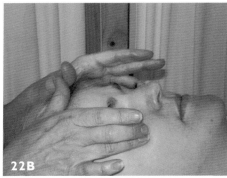

22 Make circular movements around the eyes, pausing at the inner eye, the outer corner of the eye, the centre of the eyebrow, then back to the inner corner of the eye. This movement aids the appearance of the eyes and fine lines.

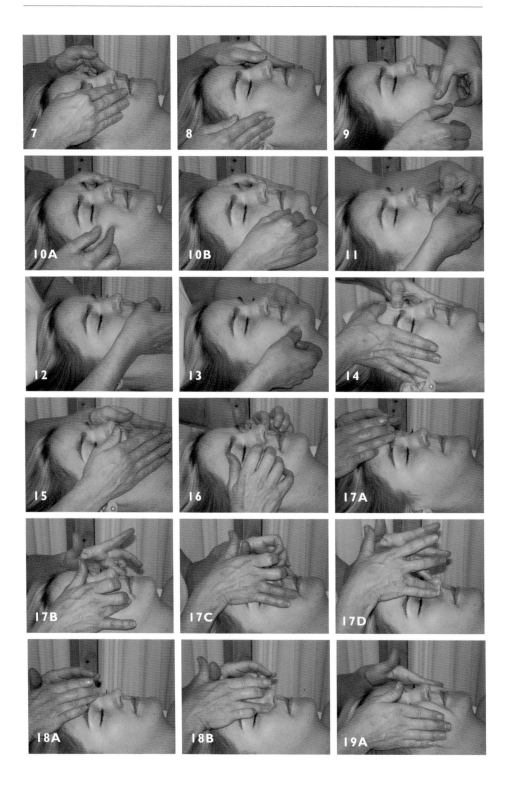

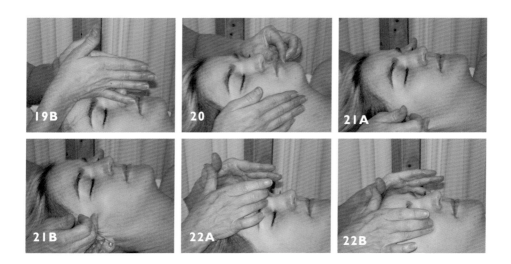

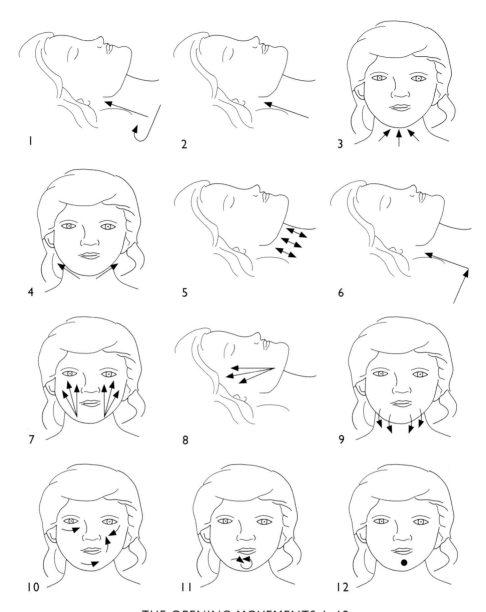

THE OPENING MOVEMENTS 1–12

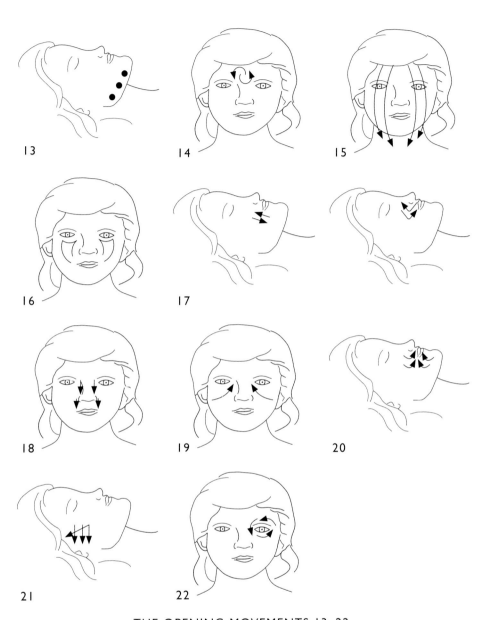

THE OPENING MOVEMENTS 13–22

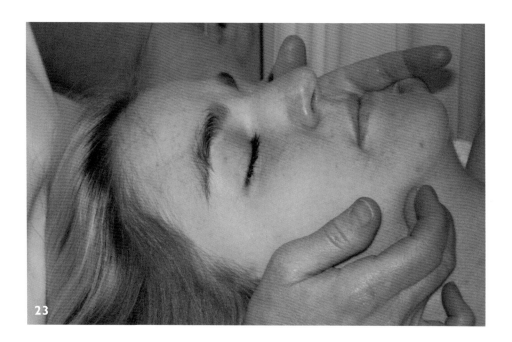

PART TWO: MERIDIAN MOVEMENTS 23–31

The following nine movements are the most important elements of this unique massage. Movements must be carried out in order, starting with the lowest acupressure point number – that is, 19 then through to 20. All acupressure points must be followed by stroking through the meridian channel using the ring or index finger.

23 Swoop up from the chin to 19, aligning with the nostrils (20). Repeat 2–3 times. Trace through the meridian channels 2–3 times.
Improves the appearance around the mouth and nose.

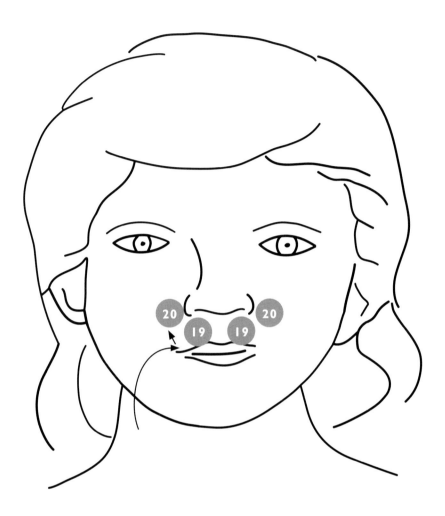

Large intestine/lung meridians: Metal

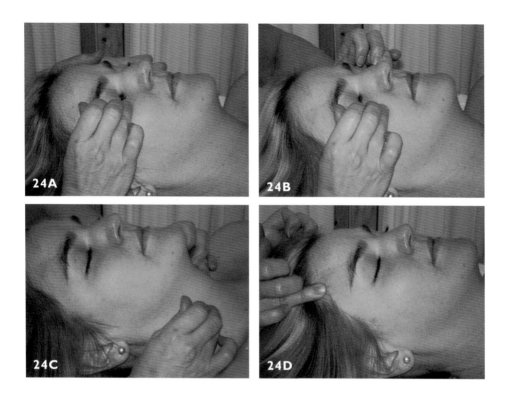

24 Rest your middle or ring finger on the bottom lashes (1). Slide the fingers down on to the small indentation of the orbit of the eye as illustrated on the following page (2), perpendicular to the nose (3), to the corner of the mouth (4), diagonally to 5, 6 and 7, up to 8, follow down to 5 and then drop down to 9. Repeat 2–3 times. Then trace through the meridian 2–3 times.

Improves appearance around the eye and the jaw.

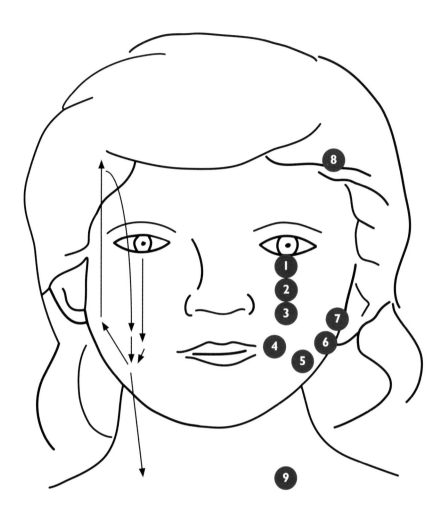

Stomach/spleen meridians: Earth

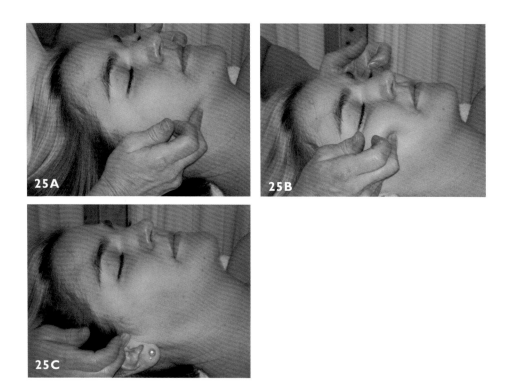

25 Find the small indentation at the mandible (jaw) (17). Follow straight up until you meet resistance at the angle of the jaw (18) and then to the middle of the ear (19).

Aids muscle firmness in this area as well as working on digestion.

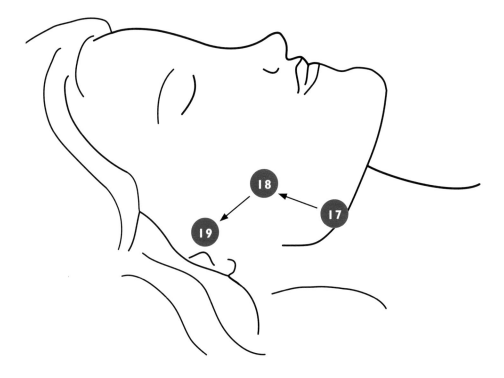

Small intestine/heart meridians: Fire

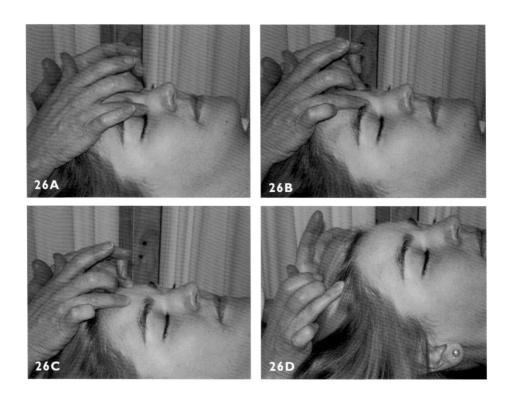

26 Rest gently at the corner of the eye (1). Follow through 2 and 3 and then out, aligned with the eye (4). Continue up for 5, 6 and 7. Improves appearance around the eyebrows and the space between.

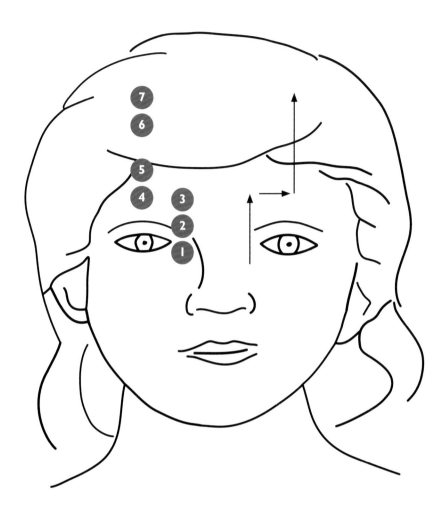

Bladder/kidney meridians: Water

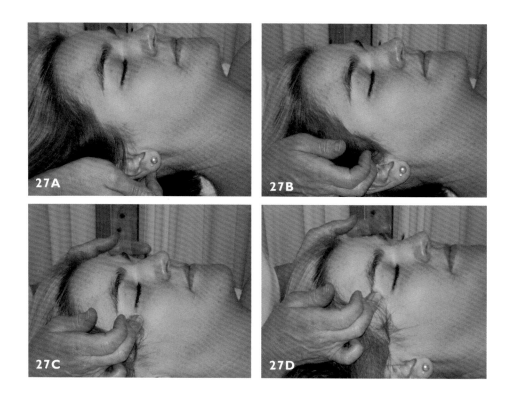

27 Sweep around from the back of the ear to the middle of the ear (1), the corner of the eye (2) and the outer edge of the eyebrow (3). Improves appearance around the eyes.

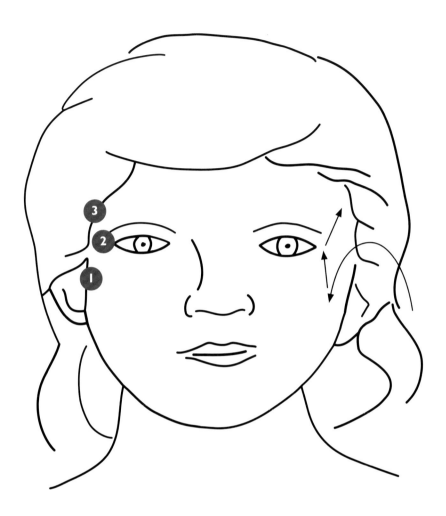

Triple heater

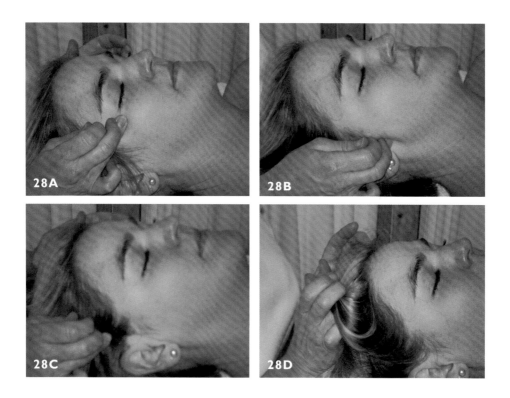

28 Start at the corner of the eye (1), down to the bottom of the ear (2), middle of the ear (3), up to the top of ear (4), then the middle top of the ear (5). Follow round the contour of the head (6, 7, 8). Sweep around perpendicular to the middle of the eye (13), straight down to the middle of the eyebrow, finding the dip on the forehead (14), just off the mid-centre line (15).

Improves the outer eyes.

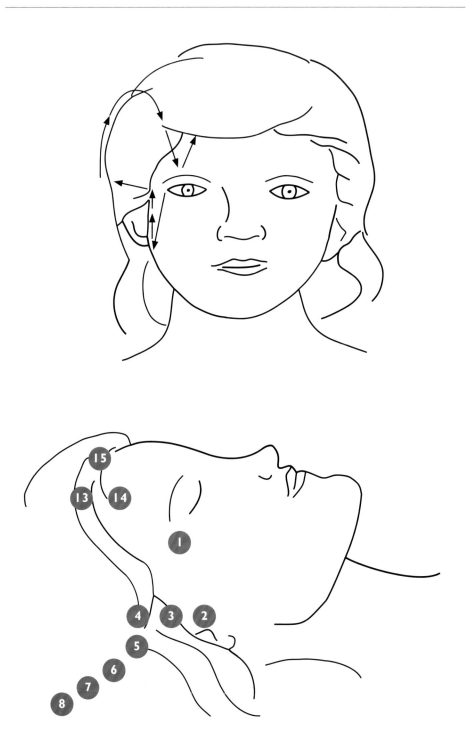

Gallbladder/liver meridians: Wood

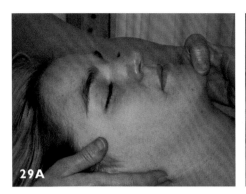 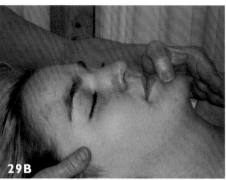

29 Find the small indentation in the centre mandible (23). Slide up to the dip in the centre of the chin (24) and then slide off the lower lip. Improves appearance and tones the chin muscles.

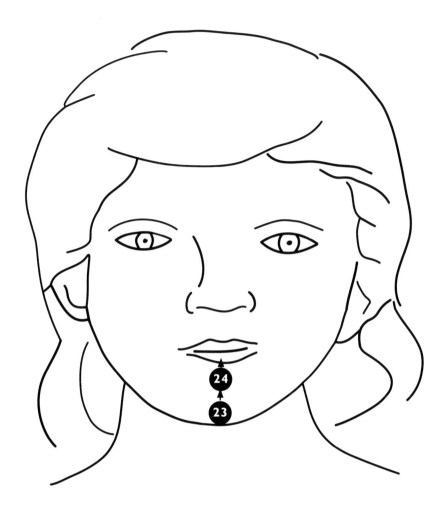

Conceptual vessel Ren Mai: Yin/Feminine

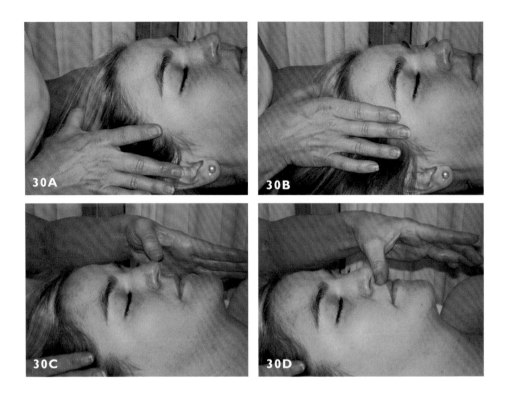

30 Find the crown point with your thumb (20), then the centre of the head (21), following down, finding the (coronal suture) just in front – a slight dip (23). Slide forwards 0.5cm (24), slide across the forehead to the top of the nose (25), down the septum to the centre of the philtrum (26) and then slide off the top lip.

Harmonises the whole body.

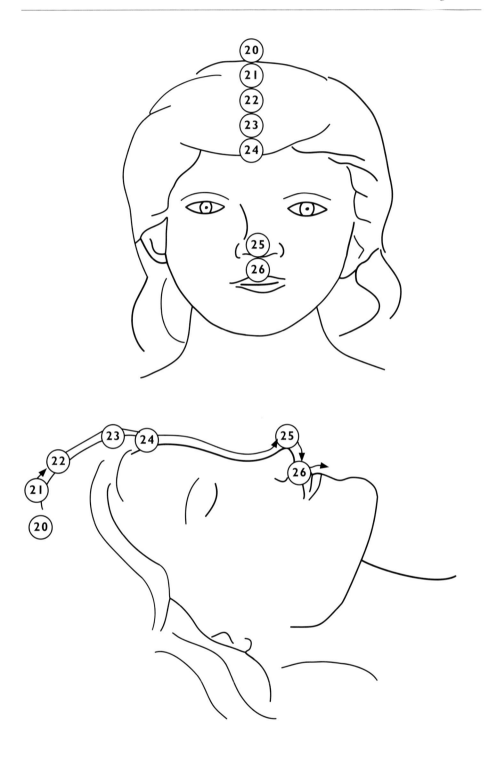

Governing vessel Du Mai: Yang/Masculine

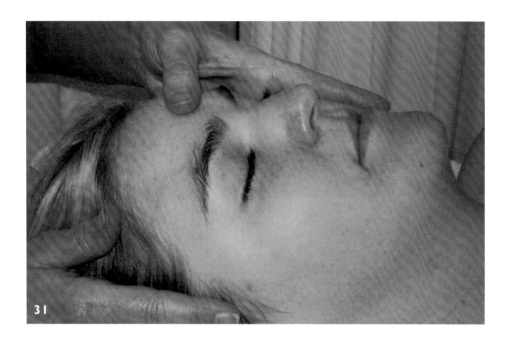

31 Place your thumb on the centre of the forehead. This balances Ki to the whole face.

Stimulates our creativity, awakens our intuition and deepens our spirituality.

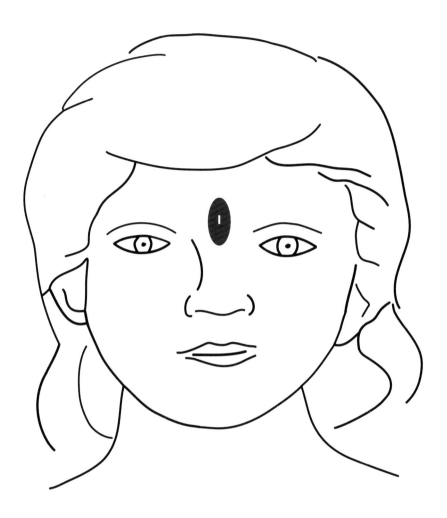

Third Eye

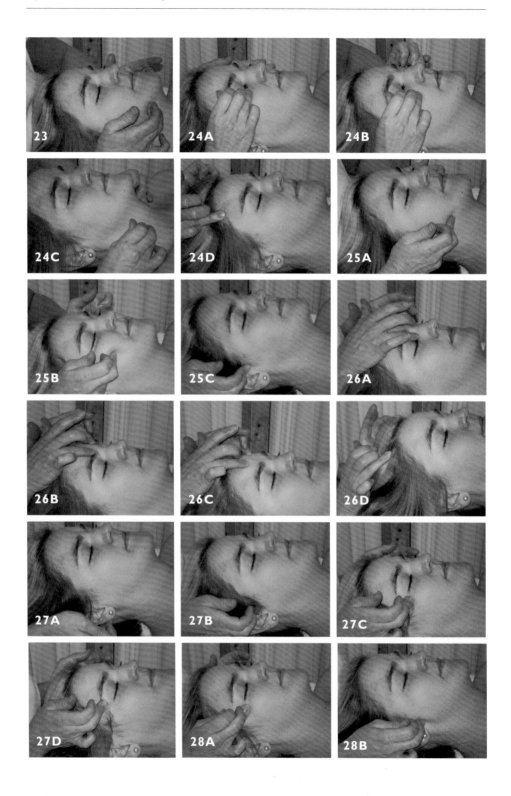

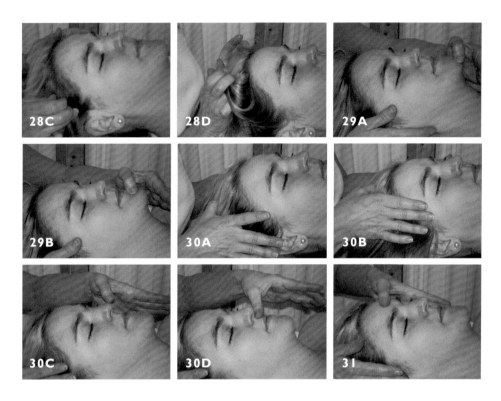

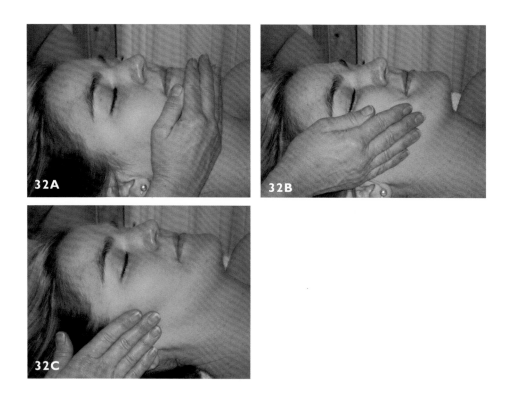

PART THREE: FINAL MOVEMENTS 32–36

32 Perform a slow effleurage movement from the chin to the cheek to the temple, in an 's' shape.

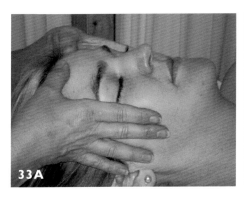 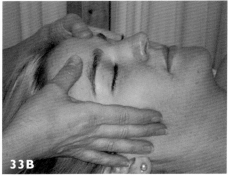

33 This is a simple drainage movement. Using your thumb, from the hairline slide towards the temples. Repeat the movement along the forehead.

Releases toxins and cellular matter back into the lymph.

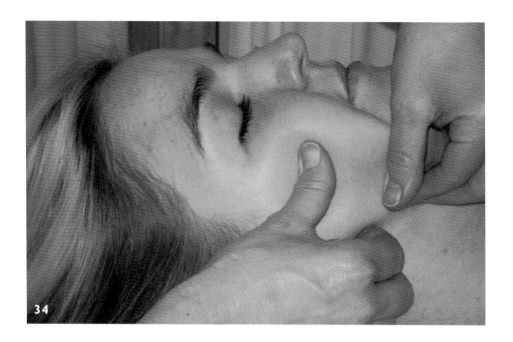

34 Perform a thumb-sliding movement. Using the side of your thumb, slide one thumb towards the chin and the second thumb towards the angle of the jaw. Repeat on the other side with medium pressure.

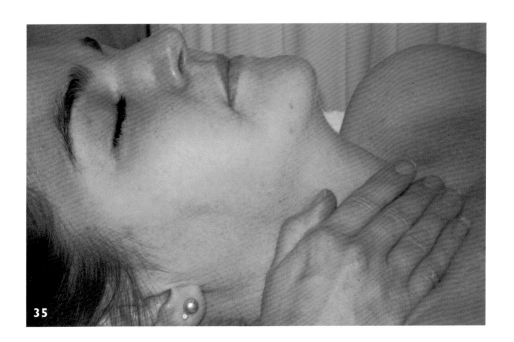

35 Perform an effleurage movement using the whole hand. Use the right hand on the right side, the left hand on the left side.
Drains lymph towards the clavicle, avoiding the oesophagus.

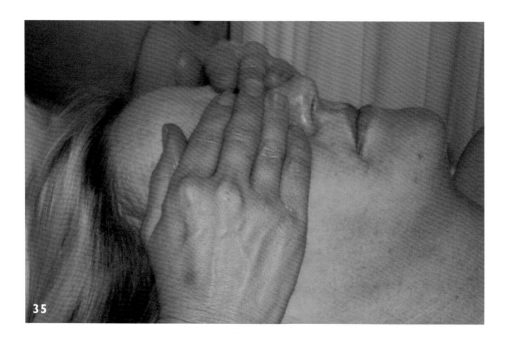

35

Closing movement

36 Apply light pressure using two fingers or the whole hand over the client's eyes, gently placing down simultaneously. Breathe three deep silent breaths to finish.

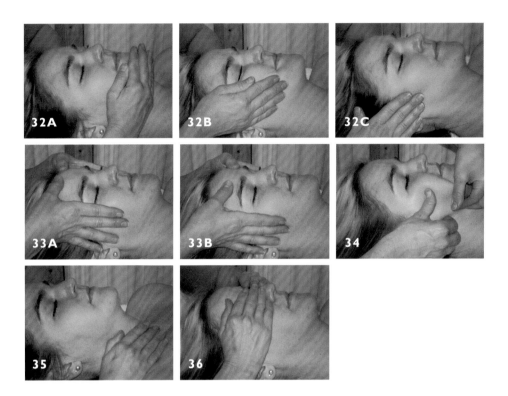

Table 6.1 The meridians

Meridian	Element	Physical	Emotional	Skincare/tone
23 Large intestine and lungs	Metal	Vitality. Constipation, diarrhoea abdominal pain, throat disorders, sinus, congestion.	Positivity. Guilt, grief, ability to accept and 'let go'. Inspiration and creativity.	Appearance around the nose and side of the mouth are improved, including fine lines. Encourages digestion, preventing blemishes, blocked pores and dull grey complexion or red mottled tone.
24 Stomach and spleen	Earth	Stillness. Oedema (bloating), flatulence, indigestion, overweight, prolapse, phlegm, cravings, perhaps ulcers.	Empathy. 'The transformer.' Assimilation – unable to accept situations. Ability to process information, intellect, being able to hold things together and put things into perspective. A preoccupation with food.	Improves the appearance around the eyes and jaw. Poor congestion may cause dull oily complexion, puffy bloated skin, especially around the eyes which will improve over time. A more defined muscle tone around the zygomaticus (cheek) and masseter (jaw) muscles.
25 Small intestine and heart	Fire	Radiates. Aids digestion and improves abdominal pain, diarrhoea, constipation, colitis, anxiety, heart problems.	Joy. 'Love and joy.' Separates pure from impure. The sorter of issues to protect the heart. Too much energy, manic. May find it hard to convey what they feel. Dull, lifeless, difficulty relating to others, absent-mindedness.	Aids muscle firmness in the jaw and cheek area. Skin can be dull, sluggish through a lack of nourishment.
26 Bladder and kidneys	Water	Understanding. Cooperates with the kidneys and endocrine system. Function is the purification of the whole body, urine and strength of teeth and bones. Urine infections, cystitis, backache, headaches, infertility, knee problems.	Fear. Worry, paranoia. The 'fight/ flight' syndrome, willpower if low, unable to respond to fear, possibly depression. May affect all other organs. Linked to the transformation of Ki.	Lifts the brows, the eye area and the space between eyes. The skin could be congested, perhaps dehydrated. Blemishes or possibly dull and lifeless with dark circles under the eyes. Responsible for the ageing process and hormonal balance.

27 Triple heater		Promotes the flow of Ki. A good energising point and controls all fluids within the body.	*Upper* heater related to chest, heart pericardium and lungs; *middle* heater to liver, gallbladder, stomach and spleen; *lower* heater to small intestines and circulation to the extremities, intestine, kidneys and bladder. Malfunction can cause oedema, palpitations, anxiety, panic, heart and digestion problems, cold hands and feet.	Aids complexion and, very importantly, is a strong boost to the immune system. Controls the spirit. A good emotional boost and helps the heart. Energising point, promotes the flow of energy and fluids that circulate throughout the body.
28 Gallbladder		The aid of hormones and secretion of bile. If neck and shoulders are very tight, then gallbladder meridian must have special attention. Coordination, digestion, gallstones, headache, nausea, eye problems.	'The decision maker.' Ability to move forward, rigidity.	Improves the edges of the eyes. Muscle tone, through tendons and ligaments, will help with double chin.
29 Extraordinary channel Ren Mai (Conceptual vessel/meridian)	Yin negative element	Controls the flow of negative Ki. Will help balance feminine Yin energy. Works on balancing hormones. Will therefore assist in all hormone-related disorders, including infertility, painful periods, menopause.	Controls the flow of negative Ki. Will help balance feminine Yin energy. Balancing right and left side of the body, restores harmony to the flow of Ki, normalising the female energies in both male and female. Intuition and nurture.	Will improve and tone the chin area. Aids skin blemishes by rebalancing hormones.
30 Extraordinary channel Du Mai (Governing vessel/ meridian)	Yang positive element	Controls the flow of positive Ki. Will help balance masculine Yang energy. Has a harmonising effect on the body, again balancing left and right side of the body. Will calm and refresh.	Good for all disorders, a powerful energiser. Again, works on hormone-related disorders including infertility.	The skin could be congested, perhaps dehydrated, with blemishes or possibly dull and lifeless with dark circles.

THE ETHOS OF NATURAL PRODUCTS

I am a keen advocate of the use of natural products not just in what I eat but also in what I use on my body – whether it is cleansing, moisturising or beautifying, I think it is an essential component of good health to use natural skincare products rather than chemically manufactured products. Being truly holistic in this sense also means understanding the energetic properties of plant extracts, plant oils and essential oils in relation to skin structure. Natural skincare products have a more long-term effect on enhancing healthy skin without the chemical build-up that can be caused by some artificial skincare products. The following is a guide to plant oils and essential oils, and their properties and usage in relation to skin type.

PLANT OILS

Plant oils used in massage are versatile and have complex healing properties, including psychological effects. They can be blended for their individual properties.

Plant oils are not just a medium within a massage sequence. The highly beneficial properties of these gentle, effective healers should be maximised beyond being an accompaniment to massage. They have a pedigree going back in time and have been used for good health, in food and for medicinal purposes. Used famously by nobility such as Cleopatra and the empresses of China for their ability to enhance and maintain beauty, plant oils are a vital part of our cosmetic and skincare regime. They are used by mixing with water, emulsifiers, waxes and gums to make cleansing lotions, balms and creams. Plant oils are essential to good health and good skin, and are contained in almost every product applied to the skin.

Table 6.2 Plant oils

Botanical oil	Properties	Skincare uses
Sweet almond (*Prunus amygdalus dulcis*)	Sweet almond is native to the Middle East, woven into the folklore of that region. For many aromatherapists, this oil is the one we turn to when giving a massage. Sweet almond is light, does not drag and mixes well with other base oils or it can be used alone. Releases tense muscle. Good for sensitive, dry, itchy skins, leaves skin feeling soft and smooth. Sweet almond contains a good amount of vitamin D, the sunshine vitamin, useful when treating the elderly or anyone recovering from illness who may lack exposure to the sun.	Used on all skin types. A good neutral oil, has no aroma, therefore useful for mixing with essential oils.
Apricot kernel (*Prunus armeniaca*)	This base oil contains laetrile or vitamin B17, said to have the ability to attack cancer cells. Although research has been inconclusive, many aromatherapists use this oil when working with cancer patients or people who are terminally ill. Usually mixed with other oils, it spreads well and is not absorbed too quickly.	It is useful for sensitive skin and dry itchy skin, and has rejuvenating properties.
Calendula (*Calendula officinalis*)	Calendula (marigold) originates from the Mediterranean and was used widely by the Egyptians. This oil is known throughout Europe as one of the best healers. Calendula can be used for inflamed skin and is a good antiseptic. It has a wonderful golden colour and is usually mixed with other base oils. Great for all skin types, especially treatment of mature or blemished skins. Calendula, with its ability to soothe and calm inflammation, will help wounds after surgery; it is used initially to relieve swelling, followed by Comfrey (see below). Calendula is a useful oil for treatment of varicose veins and thread veins within facial products. Where there is damage, redness or irritation, Calendula will help. Usually used with other base oils, not on its own.	A luxurious moisturiser or lotion, especially good for mature skins.

cont.

Table 6.2 Plant oils *cont.*

Botanical oil	Properties	Skincare uses
Comfrey *(Symphytum officinale)*	This is a marvellous oil, also steeped in folklore, used in Britain and Europe for centuries. Known as a 'cure all', its common name is Knit-bone because of its ability to heal factures and brakes. Comfrey efficiently heals bruises, and copes with muscle and ligament strains. Due to its ability to promote cell growth, it can be used after surgery, once all swelling and pain have subsided, and the wound is clean and healing normally. Comfrey is not recommended for about three months after a wound has healed and should never be used on an open wound or deep cut. Given Comfrey's ability to produce new cells, it is very useful for the treatment of varicose veins, thread veins, eczema and psoriasis. It should never be used in a whole body massage, unless mixed with other oils (use in a one-to-three ratio only).	All skin types. Particularly good on dry, mature skin, due to its ability to heal. Also wonderful for blemished skins, including acne, where the skin is rough. Especially good as a specialised mask.
Olive oil *(Olea europaea)*	Originally from the Middle East, olive oil was brought by the Moors into Spain, which is now the biggest producer of olive oil. Obtainable all over the world, millions of people utilise its properties for healing purposes. Used in balms and lotions, it nourishes and softens the skin, can be used for dry itchy skins and has anti-inflammatory properties. It is a rich oil, containing vitamins E and A, useful for the treatment of psoriasis and eczema. Relaxes aching muscles, aids circulation and is useful in the treatment of bruises and leg ulcers. It is an occlusive, which means it stays on the skin and protects against water loss; however, it can restrict the skin's ability to breathe. Olive oil has a sticky consistency and may drag. When using olive oil, ensure you always mix it with a lighter oil such as sweet almond or sunflower oil.	Good in face masks when mixed with lighter oils. Especially good on dry, sallow complexions and mature skin.

Sunflower oil *(Helianthus annuus)*	Originally from Mexico, widely used in cooking and therefore easily available, it absorbs easily into the skin. Sunflower oil has a high concentration of lecithin which helps to lower cholesterol. It has a light consistency that blends well with thicker oils, such as olive oil, suitable for dry or mature skin. Sunflower oil has an emulsifying effect, holding the oils together. When mixed with thicker oils, it will spread better on the skin, allowing it to be absorbed more easily. Recommended for oily and problem skins, due to its quick absorption rate and anti-inflammatory properties. Its high omega-6 essential fatty acid content is good for skin that bruises easily.	Very good if you wish to make your own skincare products, due to its emulsifying properties and light consistency. Mixes well.
Safflower oil *(Carthamus tinctorius)*	A member of the thistle family, with a high content of Vitamin F (omega-6). Nourishes the skin. Aids circulation in the hands and feet and is therefore good for mature skin. It has an astringent effect, helping to close large open pores. Good for making skincare products, it blends well with richer, more expensive oils.	Easily absorbed into the skin, nourishing. Good for oily skins and helps tone large pores. Blends well with almond and apricot, encouraging good blood supply and is therefore good for mature skins and enlarged pores.

ESSENTIAL OILS

Nature's little gems…a natural pharmacy…how Mother Nature really got things right…a gift from heaven to support us through joy and sorrow. There is no need to use large quantities when mixing for the individual. Essential oils sing their own song as they harmonise and penetrate in their own special way. Essential oils work on many levels, including physical, mental, emotional and spiritual. They release their power, penetrating deep into the soul, dispersing negativity with their vibrational frequencies.

Table 6.3 Essential oils

Essential oil	Properties	Skincare uses	Combinations
Rosemary (*Rosemarinus officinalis*)	Rosemary is a strong, dynamic, yet sensitive essential oil. It clears the mind, lifts the spirit and is enduring.	Good balancer. Good for oily skin yet sensitive enough to encourage vascular response in dry, sluggish complexions.	Blends with Juniper, Cypress, Basil, Lavender, Orange, Neroli.
Sandalwood (*Santalum album*)	The sheer joy of Sandalwood, sacred plant of India where the seat of so much spirituality is found, will harmonise, calm and give joy in its love of life. A luxurious essential oil used for centuries by many in the East to renew, refresh and calm.	Good for dry, mature and sensitive skin. Can also be used for acne due to its antiseptic qualities.	Blends with Cedarwood, Jasmine, Ylang Ylang.
Melissa (*Melissa officinalis*)	From this humble plant comes a dynamic essential oil that is a strong, powerful healer. It helps diminish panic and desperation, helps quieten the mind and allows you to take control of deep emotional fear.	Good for problematic skin, particularly acne.	Blends with Lemon, Lavender, Orange, Juniper.
Lavender (*Lavendula angustifolia*)	The balancer: calms the mind, quietens the soul. Always faithful, works alone or, better still, will harmonise with other essential oils. Lavender is that soothing touch, ready to do its work, neither Yin nor Yang.	Can be used for all skin types.	Blends with most oils.
Chamomile Roman (*Chamaemelum noble*)	Whenever someone needs calming, wherever there is anxiety, reach for chamomile, nature's own calmative. Allow it to sweep you on a wave of tranquillity. Calms the spirit, opens the mind and brings harmony.	Good for sensitive, fine skin, highly vascular (red), congested skin, whether oily or dry; anti-inflammatory.	Blends well with Rose, Lavender, Lemon, Orange, Juniper, Sage Clary.

Frankincense (*Boswellia carterii*)	The three wise men knew the power, strength and majesty of Frankincense – a truly wonderful healer. It simply brings you back from the abyss. Frankincense has the power to heal emotionally and physically. Definitely the one to use on inflamed skin or wounds and a must for mature skin due to its nourishing properties.	Can be used for all skin types. Especially good for congested skin. Wonderful on mature skin.	Blends well with Orange, Mandarin, Sandalwood, Lavender, Neroli, Rose, Sage Clary, Lemon.
Geranium (*Pelargonium graveolens*)	Heart of hearts, love of love, looking down. Brings joy and release from anxiety. Works well with other essential oils and powerful in its own right. It is about 'letting go'.	Works well on all skin types. Good for thread veins; astringent, balancer.	Blends well with Lavender, Orange, Sandalwood.
Neroli (*Citrus aurantium, Citrus bigaradia, Citrus vulagris*)	Stops you from falling and gives you strength during traumatic times. Nourishes. Calms the inner child, allowing you to listen to your soul.	Can be used on all skin types. Is a wonderful healer, has astringent properties and is great on mature skin.	Blends with Rosemary, Geranium, Chamomile, Lemon, Lavender, Mandarin, Orange.
Rose (*Rosa damascena, Rosa centifolia*)	The nurturer. 'Wrap your arms around me and let me feel your love. Lead me back to my path with your understanding. Allow me to find my way.' This is Rose, an empress, strong yet compassionate.	Can be used effectively on all skin types. Nourishes and aids fine lines. Lovely on its own.	Blends with Geranium, Jasmine, Lavender, Sage Clary, Chamomile.
Sage Clary (*Salvia sclarea*)	Such a good oil, its power should be revered and respected. Will lead you over troubled waters, up mountains. Brings you round to face reality with clear, wise thoughts. Shatters lack of confidence.	Good for thread veins, oily skin; astringent, stimulating.	Blends with Jasmine, Lavender, Lemon, Coriander, Rose, Sandalwood.
Jasmine (*Jasminum officinale*)	Strong, authoritative, the emperor. Will lead you with safe hands to your noble self. Allows you to have strength and confidence. Understands who you are.	Renews and rejuvenates.	Blends with Rose, Sandalwood, Ylang Ylang.

IN A NUTSHELL

- The modular nature of the facial massage routine means it can be adapted as required.

- The recipient's permission to perform the routine in medical settings is important, especially for unofficial staff such as volunteers.

- Make sure you know the recipient's history, including any reasons why this massage cannot take place.

- The setting is important: to aid the process of relaxation, ensure the recipient is warm, comfortable and away from excessive noise.

- Approach each person differently. We do not all react in the same way, so be aware of any slight responses by the recipient to your touch.

- Encourage the drinking of water to help the healing process.

- Plant and essential oils are marvellous healers. They have been used for their medicinal properties as well as part of our diet since life as we know it began. Their healing properties can be maximised for a diverse range of benefits.

- Understanding the properties of each plant oil and essential oil helps in using them for the right skin and right treatment.

- Nobility across the world, including Cleopatra and empresses of China, have used these oils for their rejuvenating properties.

Glossary

A VITAMIN: Retinol carotene is an oil-based vitamin, especially important for eyes and the immune system. It is a strong antioxidant found in fish and animal fat.

ACID MANTLE: An acidic, oily, protective layer of film on the skin, containing sebum, sweat and cellular matter.

ACNE ROSACEA: A form of acne that appears in mid-life, giving the skin a thickened, flushed appearance. There is overactivity of oily secretion, causing blemishes. The skin becomes sensitive to changes of temperature and spicy foods.

ACNE VULGARIS: A skin disorder commonly found in teenagers, affecting mainly the face. Overactivity of the oils found on the skin causes congestion, leading to blemishes, blackheads and possible inflammation.

ACUPRESSURE: A point on the surface of the skin where you can access Ki energy to harmonise the way it flows through the meridians.

ADRENALIN: A hormone produced by the adrenal glands during stress or excitement. This powerful hormone is part of the body's stress response system, commonly known as the 'fight or flight' response.

AMNA: Traditional Japanese massage.

AROMATHERAPIST: A massage therapist with extensive knowledge of the benefits of the essential oils mixed for individual circumstances and problems.

ARYANS: The name 'Aryan' describes the horse-riding, nomadic people of ancient India and ancient Iran who spoke an archaic Indo-European language. The first appearance of Aryans in history is around the middle of the second millennium BC in the Hurrian empire of Mitanni (in northern Mesopotamia). The word also means noble.

ASTRINGENT: A substance that removes excess oil from skin and usually contains alcohol.

B17 VITAMIN: Known as laetrile, which is a compound of two sugars, it has widely been researched for the treatment of cancer and is found in apricot kernels, apples, peaches, plums and cherries.

BIO-ENERGY: A natural, healing, magnetic energy field that is generated within and outside the body.

BLACKHEADS: A firm mass caused by expansion of the pores as a result of an accumulation of cellular matter and excess sebum within pores. Oxidation causes the sebum to turn black.

CAPILLARIES: Tiny blood vessels that link arteries and veins.

CELTS: A society of warriors and craftsmen who conquered much of Europe.

CHAKRA: Sanskrit word meaning 'wheel', it describes the spinning vortex of energy centres in and around the body. The seven main chakras or energy centres affect our physical, emotional, mental and spiritual well-being.

CHLOASMA: Pigmentation of the skin caused by overactivity of melanin cells. Commonly found during pregnancy.

CLAVICLE: A long bone of the chest, commonly known as the collar bone.

COLLAGEN: The connective tissue of the dermis. It is a soluble substance that gives skin its soft, full appearance but which deteriorates with age, becoming rigid and unable to retain fluids.

COMEDONE: A firm mass which causes an expansion of the pores as a result of an accumulation of cellular matter and excess sebum within the pores. Oxidation of the sebum causes the sebum to turn black. Commonly known as blackheads.

CONFUCIANISM: A philosophy and way of life based on a respect for nature founded by Confucius, a Chinese thinker, political figure and educator who did not believe in an afterlife.

CORONAL SUTURE: The line of junctions of the frontal bone with two parietal bones of the cranium.

CTM: Chinese Traditional Medicine.

D VITAMIN: Known as calciferol, vesterol, ergosterol. Commonly known as the sunshine vitamin because it is processed by the liver from sunshine. It is also found in some cereals and promotes healthy bones and teeth.

DEMULCENT: An agent or substance that forms a soothing or protective coating. Demulcents on the skin can be moisturising, cooling or hydrating.

DERMIS: The second or middle layer of skin. It is 10–40 times deeper than the epidermis and is made up of blood vessels, lymph vessels, elastin, collagen and water. Hair follicles and sweat glands are also located in the dermis and together they help to regulate temperature and aid the healing process.

DIS-EASE: A state of disruption to the physical, emotional, mental or spiritual body of a person when they are not in harmony or at ease with their higher self or divine consciousness.

DIVINE: A higher power. It is a spiritual and natural concept describing the omnipotent, universal life force. This is the source or origin of all life and creation.

DRUIDS: Druids are considered teachers, ritualists, counsellors and shamans. They practise Druidry which is one of the earliest native spiritual movements across Britain and Europe. It is thought to have developed almost 3000 years ago during the European Iron Age, although some believe it has been around much longer than that. Druids are pagans who believe in connecting with the cycles of life, spirits of nature, ancestors and ancestral gods for life in balance with the universe and nature.

E vitamin: Known as tocopherol, a strong antioxidant, anti-ageing and anticoagulant found in wheatgerm, wholegrain cereals and soya beans.

Effleurage: A smooth rhythmic massage movement using the whole flat of the hand.

Elastin: A protein found in the skin and tissue of the body. It has a spring coil-like property within the elastic fibres of connective tissue and it accounts for the elasticity of structures such the skin, blood vessels, heart, lungs, intestines, tendons and ligaments. It helps to keep skin flexible but tight, providing a bounce-back reaction if the skin is pulled. It also helps to keep skin smooth as it stretches to accommodate normal activities such as flexing a muscle or opening and closing the mouth to talk or eat.

Element: A charge or vibration of energy.

Emollient: A substance made from oils and water.

Emulsifiers: A substance that separates oils from water.

Endorphins: Neurotransmitters found in the brain and pituitary gland and other parts of the body. Similar to morphine, endorphins are produced as a response to stimuli such as stress, fear or pain. The neurotransmitters interact with receptor cells found in regions of the brain responsible for blocking pain and controlling emotion.

Epidermis: The upper layer of the skin consisting of several layers of flattened cells (squamous cells). The deepest part of the epidermis has melanocytes, the cells that produce melanin and give skin its colour.

Essential oil: A concentrated oil containing chemical compounds with therapeutic properties, extracted from plants, usually by expression (pressure) or by steam.

F vitamin: Unsaturated fatty acid, essential for life. Produces prostaglandins, hormone-like substances vital to life. Found in nuts, seeds and avocado.

Fight or flight syndrome: Commonly used to describe the action of the autonomic nervous system, a primitive reaction to stress.

Galen: Claudius Galenus is considered to be the greatest philosopher, physician and herbalist of ancient Rome. He developed the teachings of the Greek philosopher Hippocrates from which early Western medicine evolved.

Grounding: Maintaining the connection to the earth to remain focused and clear of thought.

Hinduism: A religious, philosophical and cultural practice that originated in India. Hindus believe in reincarnation, one absolute being of multiple manifestations, and the law of cause and effect (among many other beliefs).

Hormones: Chemical messengers, transmitting signals to various areas to ensure smooth bodily functions.

Insertion of the muscle: Where the muscle attaches to the bone, skin or surface fascia, which relaxes during movement.

Ki: Japanese name for healing life force energy, a vibrational healing energy found in all living things, including the earth and the universe.

LYMPHATIC SYSTEM: A subsidiary circulatory system of lymphatic vessels lying close to blood capillaries, which flood the muscles and body tissues with a fluid called lymph. Lymph is rich in nutrient and antibodies, produced by cells found in lymph nodes. Part of the immune system.

MANDIBLE: Lower jaw bone.

MASSETER: A rectangular muscle of mastication that aids the action of closing the jaw.

MEDITATION: A form of deep relaxation that allows the body and the brain to rest.

MELANIN: A dark pigmentation of the skin produced by cells called melanocytes. Exposure to the sun stimulates production of melanin which protects the skin against burning.

MENTALIS: A small triangular muscle of the chin which elevates the lower lip, causing wrinkling of the chin.

MERIDIAN: Known in Chinese Traditional Medicine as an invisible channel or pathway that runs throughout the body, flowing from the lung/large bowel to the gallbladder/liver.

MILIA: A solid mass of sebum that becomes trapped in the sebaceous duct. Commonly known as a whitehead.

MUSCLE ORIGIN: Where the muscle attaches to the bone, skin or surface fascia, which is fixed during movement.

NAKHEBET: The vulture goddess of ancient Egypt, the mother god. Symbolises recreation.

OCCIPITAL: One of the seven bones of the cranium, found at the base.

OMEGA-6: An essential fatty acid which makes prostaglandins, a hormone-like substance vital to life.

OESOPHAGUS: Carries food from the mouth to the stomach. Also known as the gullet.

PETRISSAGE: A compression movement applied to the skin and muscles. The action of compression and relaxation brings a vascular response, flooding the area with nutrients and releasing tense muscles, thereby benefiting the skin.

PRANA: The ancient Yogic term for the subtle healing energy thought to be taken in during breathing.

PROCERUS: A narrow muscle attached to the nasal bone, between the eyebrows.

QI: Chinese name for healing life force energy, a vibrational healing energy found in all living things, including the earth and the universe.

SANSKRIT: An ancient Indo-Aryan language, regarded as the liturgical language of Hinduism, Buddhism and Jainism. It is currently one of the 22 official languages of India. The word 'Sanskrit' means refined, consecrated or sanctified.

SCAPULA: A large triangular bone known, commonly as the shoulder blade.

SEBUM: An oily secretion that protects the skin from bacteria and helps to maintain a supple, smooth complexion.

SENSORY NERVES: Nerves that pass impulses from the receptors towards or to the central nervous system. They let the brain know if something feels hot, cold, smooth or rough, and so on.

SHAKTI: A mythological figure, the divine cosmic female power, without form. According to yogic tradition, Shakti lies dormant in all beings, like a coiled spring ready to be released.

SHINTO: Literally means 'way of the gods' (Shen Tao in Chinese). Shinto is the indigenous religion of Japan that venerates nature and animals.

SHIVA: A mythological figure, the divine cosmic male power, pure manifestation of consciousness, without form. Sometimes known as the destroyer.

SUFISM: Considered to be the inner, mystical or spiritual dimension of Islam. The central tenet of Sufism is purity of the heart through total submission to God's will. It is thought that one of the original meanings of the word 'Sufi' is 'purity'.

TAOISM: The ancient religion and philosophy of China. Tao means the way, path or principle. Central beliefs are the importance of the harmonisation of one's will with nature and that everything has a purpose.

TAPOTEMENT: A percussion movement using light tapping which stimulates a nervous response.

TONE: A term used to describe the tension of the muscle. For example, high tone means strong tension, possibly leading to fatigued muscles or flaccid lack of tension.

TSUBO: Japanese word for acupressure point.

UATCHET: The snake goddess who symbolised protection and fertility. Together with Nakhebet, became the symbol on the crowns of Egypt, over the Third Eye.

VITILIGO: Lack of pigmentation on the skin. Small white patches appearing on the face or body may join together to make larger areas that are sensitive to the sun's rays.

WHITEHEAD: A solid mass of sebum that becomes trapped in the sebaceous duct. Also known as milia.

YANG: The masculine opposite and complement to Yin; energy that flows in a downward spiral from the universe.

YELLOW EMPEROR: The author of the classic book of medicine Huang Di Nei Jing Su Wen, the Yellow Emperor, or Huang Di, ruled China towards the end of the third century BC. He was credited with numerous inventions and innovations, and was considered a cosmic ruler and patron of esoteric arts. His rule was defined by the creation of the Huang Di Nei Jing Su Wen, upon which much of Chinese Traditional Medicine is based.

YIN: The feminine opposite and complement to Yang; energy that flows upwards from the earth.

YOGI: A person who links with the Divine through meditation and the physical postures of yoga, leading to enlightenment and being at one with the Divine.

ZYGOMATIC: Also known as the zygomaticus major, part of a set of muscles found in the cheekbones. Extending from the top of the cheekbone to the corners of the mouth, it functions during facial expressions such as laughing, smiling or wincing.

Bibliography and Further Reading

Allan, V. (2006) *Ocean of Streams: Zen Shiatsu – Meridians, Tsubos and Theoretical Impressions*. Thornhill: Omki.

Arewa, C.S. (2001) *Way of Chakras*. London: Thorsons.

Borseth, K. (2008) *The Aromantic Guide to Making Your Own Natural Skin, Hair and Body Care Products*. Moray: Aromantic.

Borseth, K. (2008) *The Aromantic Guide to Unlocking the Powerful Health and Rejuvenating Benefits of Vegetable Oils*. Moray: Aromantic.

Brennan, B.A. (1987) *Hands of Light: A Guide to Healing Through the Human Energy Field*. New York, NY: Bantam Books.

Brown, S. (2008) *Face Reading: Secrets of the Chinese Masters*. New York, NY: Sterling Publishing.

Firebrace, P. and Hill, S. (1994) *A Guide to Acupuncture*. London: Hamlyn.

Gach, M.R. (1992) *Acupressure: How to Cure Common Ailments the Natural Way*. London: Piatkus Books.

Gallant, A. (1987) *Principles and Techniques for the Beauty Specialist* (2nd Edition). Cheltenham: Stanley Thornes.

Hicks, A. (2005) *The Acupuncture Handbook: How Acupuncture Works and How It Can Help You*. London: Piatkus Books.

Judith, A. (1987) *Wheels of Life: The Classic Guide to the Chakra System*. Woodbury, MN: Llewellyn Publications.

Kushi, M. (2007) *Your Body Never Lies: The Complete Book of Oriental Diagnosis*. New York, NY: Square One Publishers.

Liechti, E. (1998) *The Complete Illustrated Guide to Shiatsu: The Japanese Healing Art of Touch for Health and Fitness*. Dorset: Elements Books.

McKenzie, E. (2001) *Healing Reiki: Reunite Mind, Body and Spirit with Healing Energy*. London: Hamlyn.

Saeki, C. (2004) *The Japanese Skincare Revolution: How to Have the Most Beautiful Skin of Your Life – At Any Age*. Tokyo: Kodansha International.

Stux, G., Berman, B. and Pomeranz, B. (2003) *Basics of Acupuncture* (5th Edition). Berlin: Springer Medizin Verlag.

Wilson, K.J. (1963) *Ross and Wilson Anatomy and Physiology*. London: E & S Livingstone.

Worwood, V.A. (1999) *The Fragrant Heavens: The Spiritual Dimension of Fragrance and Aromatherapy*. Novato, CA: New World Library.

Useful Websites

For courses in Japanese Holistic Face Massage held in the UK and internationally

Rosemary Patten

Equinox Rose

www.equinoxrose.com

For courses in making your own skincare products

Kolbjorn Borseth

Aromantic

www.aromantic.co.uk

Suppliers of essential oils and skincare material

G Baldwin & Co

www.baldwins.co.uk

Materia Aromatica

www.materiaaromatica.com

Aromantic

www.aromantic.co.uk